Dr. Martina Zangger has a PhD specialising in the field of inter-personal violence and a Master's Degree in Couple and Family Therapy. She has worked at the frontline helping women and children impacted by sexual assault and domestic violence for more than 20 years. Using a holistic, trauma-informed, feminist practice model, she assists traumatised clients to find safety and healing.

Martina has worked for over a decade as a university lecturer helping medical students to become patient-centred communi-cators and empathic practitioners. She teaches students to provide a compassionate, non-judgemental response to their patients. Now, as an Honorary Lecturer, she provides guest lectures on sexuality, diversity, social justice and mental health.

Her PhD focuses on sexual assault and the legal system. She has presented her PhD research 'Women of Courage' at confer-ences in Australia and overseas.

Martina divides her time between Awabakal (Newcastle) and Woromi Lands (Forster). She is a passionate feminist and social justice advocate, and an introvert who loves reading, napping, knitting, tapestry, and spending time with her family, women friends and in nature. Trees are her inspiration, teaching her to remain steady in stormy weathers, with roots deep inside Mother Earth. Her partner and their twenty-six-year-old daughter surround her with deep love and unwavering support.

NOT MY SHAME

A Memoir

Martina Zangger

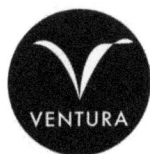

VENTURA

First published in 2025 by Ventura Press
PO Box 780, Edgecliff NSW 2027 AUSTRALIA
www.venturapress.com.au

Not My Shame
ISBN 978-1-7638320-5-3 (Print book)
ISBN 978-1-7638320-7-7 (ebook)

Cover: Deborah Parry Graphics
Internal Design: Luke Harris, WorkingType Books

A catalogue record for this
book is available from the
National Library of Australia

Ventura Press acknowledges the Traditional Owners of the country on which
we work, the Gadigal people of the Eora nation, and recognises their continuing
connection to the land, waters and culture. We pay our respects to their Elders past,
present and emerging.

I want those women to say,
Mrs Pelicot did it, we can do it too.
I don't want them to feel shame.
When you're raped there is shame.
But it's not for us to have shame.
It's for them.
Shame must change sides.
Gisèle Pelicot

Make peace
with all the women
you once were.

lay flowers
at their feet.

offer them incense
and honey
and forgiveness.

Emory Hall

This work was written on the unceded lands of the First Nations peoples. I honour their enduring connection to Country, storytelling, and culture. I am grateful to live and write on this land, and I pay my deep respects to Elders past, present, and emerging.

A Note to the Reader:

This is a story of survival and healing, but it includes references to sexual violence and other traumatic experiences. I offer this warning with care, knowing that some readers may need to approach certain parts with caution or skip them entirely. Please take care of yourself as you read.

PROLOGUE

April 2025

The Taoists say that each human life holds ten thousand joys and ten thousand sorrows. No one is exempt, and our sorrows will come to us all. Mine began in early childhood and continued into adolescence and my twenties. In order to discover my joys, I had to first find the courage to wade thigh-deep through the muck of long-buried traumas. I had to face the consequences of the reckless decisions I made as a young woman. In my mid-twenties, I was fortunate to discover the profound transformation that occurs in the sanctity of the therapy room. Gradually, I learned to hold my sorrows gently in the palms of my hands, like tiny baby birds, with infinite patience and kindness. And much later, the joys came to me, like precious jewels.

Raised in an authoritarian household in Switzerland, I experienced sexual abuse in early childhood at the hands of my maternal grandfather, a prominent judge and academic, and my maternal uncle, a highly regarded Swiss politician. I didn't stand a chance against the further abuses I experienced. For decades I believed I was a magnet for perverts, that the sexual violence I suffered was somehow my fault. It took years of therapy to become a strong woman with boundaries, able to have a voice and put the blame where it belongs. The abuse is not my shame, but that of the perpetrators who chose to harm me.

As I complete the final edits of this story, a familiar fear invades me, like large brown moths beating their wings inside my stomach.

Sleep eludes me. My story will be in the public realm and people will judge me. Family, colleagues and even strangers will think of me as a moral delinquent, unhinged and 'psycho'. I hear my mother's familiar voice. Even though she is long dead, she still has the power to berate me in her harsh Swiss German.

How dare you reveal our secrets! You are sullying our family's good name, she hisses. The Swiss must keep family dysfunction hidden behind lace-curtained windows and locked doors.

I remind myself not to listen to my mother. Instead, I celebrate the achievement of sharing my life story, just like when I received my PhD titled 'Women of Courage'. Gently, I hold the tiny birds of fear in the palms of my hands. Softly, I kiss the tops of their delicate feathered heads. Taking slow deep breaths, I put my hands over my heart and whisper to myself, *I'm proud of you.* These words of self-compassion liberate me from the shame that is not mine to carry, allowing me to release my story into the world.

This is the story as I have lived it, as it has echoed in my memory and settled in the quiet spaces of my heart. It is, unavoidably, a subjective account – shaped by the passage of time, the haze of emotion, and the imperfect lens through which we all view our past. I do not claim to speak for anyone else. This is my truth, told as honestly as I can, knowing that others may remember differently. And that, too, is part of the story. To protect those who may not wish to be part of this telling, I have changed some names and details. Their presence is still felt; their identities are simply veiled.

PART ONE:
FALLING

CHAPTER ONE

1981

Rajneesh, dressed in a white kaftan, gazes at me from a large, framed photo on the wall opposite my bed. His eyes twinkle – bottomless, dark and liquid. His white beard, long hair and gentle face beckon me towards a brand-new spiritual life. I hold my hands in front of my heart in the namaste prayer, the traditional Hindu salute of reverence.

Aged nineteen, I've become one of Rajneesh's one hundred thousand devotees after reading his book, *My Way, The Way of the White Clouds*. My adoration of him is the profoundest form of love I've felt for anyone in my short life. I've spent days dying my clothes red, orange, purple and pink – the shades of the rising sun and the colours worn by Rajneesh's devotees. Wearing my new mala, a sandalwood necklace, I gaze at the locket containing a photograph of my Indian guru. I love the Sanskrit spiritual name Rajneesh has bestowed on me, *Pragito*. Reborn as a completely new person with a new name, I'm free from a past. Inserting a cassette – one of his sermons – into the cassette recorder, I press play and listen to his voice. It's as though he's speaking directly to me, his honey-toned words and lilting accent mesmerising.

'Surrender to me and I will transform you. That is my promise.' Each sentence ends with his signature drawn-out last letter, its effect hypnotic. 'Meditation is the way to stop the very idea of time as fluuuux. Meditation is a total stillnesss. Nothing mooooves.'

Sitting cross-legged on my futon, I place the palms of my hands on my heart, his words filling me with a profound longing. Certain I've discovered my life's purpose, I resolve to devote myself completely to him and to a spiritual life. If I save enough money, I'll soon be living with him on his sixty-four-thousand-acre desert ashram in America. I picture myself kneeling at his feet and bowing down before him in devotion. All I need to do is save up eight thousand dollars so that I can stay with him for a whole year and reach the enlightenment he's promised those fortunate enough to appreciate his holiness.

I now have three names: Martina, the name my parents gave me and which I have rejected; Pragito, meaning 'Song of Love', the name my guru has given me; and Zoe, the sexy new call-girl name that I'll be using to earn money the quickest way possible. I'll be working my first shift tonight at Penthouse, an upmarket brothel in Sydney's business district. As I sit on the futon, I wonder whether there is an incongruity between being a call girl and a spiritual seeker. But I quickly decide the idea that sex work is immoral is a social construct that doesn't apply to me now that I've embarked on a spiritual path. I reason it's okay to be a sex worker *and* a spiritual seeker because I no longer have to obey the rules that society and my authoritarian parents have imposed on me.

But soon, Mum's thick Swiss German voice hisses inside my head, *You've gone completely mad. You're in love with a bogus guru you've never even met!* Mum will disown me if she finds out about my new job, but I quickly banish this thought. I love Rajneesh, and I'm willing to do anything to be with him. Surely, it's a spiritual act to surrender wholeheartedly to one's guru.

I go to the bathroom to prepare for tonight's shift. I stand under the shower and shave my legs, underarms and bikini line with the new razor I bought at the corner shop. I haven't removed my body hair since I became a hippie in my mid-teens. I lather soap and hot water onto my legs and begin to shave the thick pelt of hair. I watch as the long brown hairs swirl in a circle at the bottom of the shower and then disappear down the drain. Next, I shave my underarms and bikini line. When I step out of the shower and dry my body, I admire its sexy sleekness. I rub Nivea cream into my smooth skin and put on my new red lacy g-string and bra, a pink skirt and a purple crop top.

§

At five in the afternoon, I climb onto my red pushbike in Darlinghurst, ride into town past the Ferrari showroom on William Street, then up the hill past St Mary's Cathedral and finally arrive at Penthouse on Pitt Street in the heart of the city. Carrying the bike up the steep, dark stairs, I enter the reception area out of breath. My hands shake with fear of the strangers I'll have to have sex with tonight. I don't even know if I'm any good at sex. I worry the clients won't want me, an awkward, chubby teenager. Paul, my new boss, has red pitted acne scars. His intense blue eyes are friendly and his carefully tended dark curls make me think he might be gay.

'Hi Paul, I was here for my interview yesterday. I'm supposed to start at six.' My voice is shaky, revealing my lack of confidence.

'Ah yes, Zoe, come with me. I'll show you around,' Paul says, smiling. 'This is the lounge room where you'll be relaxing in between clients.'

I wave hello to half a dozen women sitting around on white couches in front of the television. They are smoking, drinking champagne and painting their nails. Next, we walk into a large room with cement flooring, a wall of mirrors, a row of grey metal lockers and four shower stalls.

'You'll shower here in between clients and do your make-up. This is your locker.' Paul hands me a key.

What have I done? My stomach fills with a rush of panic and my hands shake.

'You'll be okay, Zoe.' Paul gives my shoulder a squeeze. He can probably sense my fear.

I put my bag in the locker and follow Paul up the stairs to the second floor. He opens the door to one of the rooms. It has no windows and is dimly lit by a bedside lamp and I'm immediately claustrophobic. There's a king-sized bed with red satin sheets and two fluffy white towels folded in the shape of a swan. I wonder whether I'll have to learn to fold towels into swans.

'This is your room, where you'll be looking after your clients tonight,' Paul says. Stevie Wonder's 'Isn't She Lovely' is playing in the background. Paul picks up the alarm clock and shows me how to set it for either thirty minutes or an hour, depending on the service the client has booked. He shows me the large red button on the wall next to the door.

'You can press this duress alarm in case one of them gets nasty.'

My heart thumps a fast rhythm inside my chest. 'Do they become nasty?' I ask, wide-eyed.

'Only sometimes, but you'll be okay,' Paul says reassuringly as he pats my shoulder.

I quickly push my fear out of my mind and conjure up a string of kind, handsome men who will shower me with tips.

We walk upstairs to the rooftop, where there are several blue-lit round spas.

'You'll relax here with your clients while they chill out with a beer or champagne after a stressful day at work.'

We return downstairs to the locker room, where Paul hands me my uniform, a skimpy white dress. He introduces me to Donna, a busty woman in her thirties with long legs and a shiny black bob. Her dark brown eyes are almond shaped, and she's busy attaching her black lace stockings to a suspender belt.

Paul introduces us. 'Donna, this is Zoe, it's her first shift tonight.'

Donna puts an arm around me and smiles warmly. I'm sure she can see my trembling hands.

'You'll be all right, love. Go and get changed and then I'll help you do your make-up.'

My uniform barely covers my knickers: a soft white tunic split from top to bottom on both sides, secured with a wide red belt that pairs with the new red patent-leather stilettos and lacy g-string and bra. During our interview yesterday, Paul took one look at my saggy cotton undies and hairy legs and shook his head sadly. He recommended I shave my legs and purchase some lingerie from the House of Merivale, an upmarket boutique just a few doors from Penthouse. When I entered the shop, I felt immediately out of place and my new purchases cost me nearly all the money in my Commonwealth Bank account.

This afternoon in the locker room, my sexy new underwear and stilettoes provide me with a small amount of confidence as I gaze at myself in the floor-to-ceiling mirror. Taking a seat in front of the mirror on one of the white fluffy stools, I pull down my tiny dress to cover my dimply thighs while I contemplate my face that looks grey, my pupils large with fear. By now, I'm truly terrified and my former bravado has left me altogether.

Mum hisses at me inside my head, *I'm ashamed of you. You look like a slut!*

'You're very pale, Zoe. I'm going to bring some colour to your face.' Donna gathers her boxes, tubes and potions of make-up.

Being a new age girl, the only thing I'm familiar with is eyeliner.

The soft caressing movement of Donna's brush soothes my fear as I surrender to her touch.

'Now we'll put on some eye shadow and false eye lashes to frame your beautiful blue eyes.'

Donna's motherly touch is deeply soothing and I want to sit there forever. I don't want to have sex with strange men.

Donna applies a deep red lipliner and lipstick. She adds a soft shade of rouge to my cheeks and blends it with her fingers. Mum wasn't any good at affection, so the longing for tenderness has been a constant companion in my life. Donna dabs some of her Chanel No 5 perfume on my neck, between my breasts and behind my ears.

'Have a look, you're stunning. You'll break some hearts tonight, girl.' Donna smiles.

I open my eyes and a mysterious young woman stares back at me. I look five years older and like a real woman.

'Thank you, Donna. You're so lovely to help me.' I squeeze her hand.

'Come meet the others,' she says, putting lip gloss on her full lips.

We walk into the staff lounge, where half a dozen women sit on two large white faux-leather sofas, smoking cigarettes. The women are drinking Yellowglen champagne from plastic flutes.

'Everyone, this is Zoe. It's her first shift, so be nice to her.' Donna takes a seat on one of the sofas.

The women smile at me as I perch on the edge of one of the sofas. My legs pump up and down with nervous energy, and I pick at my cuticles. One of them begins to bleed, and I quickly hide it in the palm of my hand. Everyone is confident and beautiful, while I feel frumpy in my small white dress. I look down at my thighs. They are too thick and they stick to the vinyl couch while *Sale of the Century* blares on the television. Lighting a cigarette, I take a deep drag to calm myself. At least the tightly belted tunic shows off my small waist and large breasts. I've never worn a g-string before. It creeps uncomfortably between my butt cheeks, and I pull it out when I hope no one is looking.

§

Half an hour later, Paul introduces me to Alistair, my first client. He is a tall, lanky, grey-haired man in his early forties, wearing thick glasses, a dark blue suit, starched white shirt and red tie. The two of us walk upstairs together to my room. My stilettos are already uncomfortable, and a large blister has formed on my right heel. I open the door to the room, unsure what to do next. I hide my fear by giving Alistair a wide fake smile. I glance at the red duress alarm, the basket of condoms, the large tub of KY Jelly and the bottle of Johnson's Baby Oil on the bedside table. I remain close to the door, ready to flee. Alistair pulls me into his chest, my body rigid. He smells of expensive aftershave.

'How long have you been working here, Zoe?'

'Not long, but I've already learned a lot,' I lie. 'What service would you like?' I sound ridiculous.

'I just want to spend time with a beautiful girl like you, so I can forget all my worries for an hour.' He slowly removes my belt and dress and gazes at me. 'Oh my, you are lovely,' he sighs.

I smile, relieved he thinks I'm good enough. I pull in my stomach to make my waist appear smaller.

'Have a shower, and then we'll have some fun,' I say, trying to appear confident. But deep inside my stomach, I'm cold and scared.

Alistair undresses, hangs his suit, shirt and tie onto coat hangers, and steps into the shower. Taking a peek at his long, thin penis, I'm suddenly terrified that I'll have to have sex with him. Setting the clock for an hour the way Paul showed me, I apply a large dollop of

KY Jelly and lie on the bed trying out my most seductive pose as I wait for Alistair to join me.

He towels himself dry and lies down next to me. Soon, he's inside me. As I lie beneath him, I focus on the ornate art deco ceiling and think about the money I'm earning. I moan using a fake sexy voice. But soon I start to worry that the condom might break. I could end up pregnant or catch a disease.

'Oh, what a special treat this is for me, Zoe. My wife is menopausal, and she hates sex,' he confides as he pushes deeper inside me and gazes at me with tender eyes. Suddenly, he starts to slam his penis into me, hard and fast. Every thrust hurts and, desperate for him to finish, I moan louder and dig my nails into his back in a pretend fit of passion. Finally, the ordeal is over and he lies down beside me, out of breath. When he strokes my face, his hands are soft.

'Thank you, Zoe. That was wonderful. You're going to be my special little secret. My wife spends all the money I earn on my Mastercard, as if money grows on trees, and my three teenage kids don't respect me.' Alistair sighs.

I think about needing to find a Band-Aid for my blister while I tickle Alistair's back until the alarm goes off. When I give him a kiss goodbye, I decide that my new job is easy.

That night, I provide a service to four more men. At three in the morning, feeling proud of all the cash in my backpack, I ride home on my pushbike. My vagina is sore as I sit on the bike's seat and cycle up William Street past the Coca-Cola sign at Kings Cross and back to my share house in Darlinghurst.

CHAPTER TWO

Three months earlier
1981

When I arrive at Gaya, a commune on the south coast of New South Wales, my boyfriend Tim flings open the car door, picks me up and swings me round and round in wide circles on the vivid green lawn. We laugh and kiss deeply and when he puts me down, I notice he is wearing torn pyjama bottoms, without underpants, and a dirty-looking white-grey Bonds singlet. His bum crack shows, and I try hard to ignore the body odour emanating from him. I don't want to appear petty, since living on a commune means rejecting conventional values, including daily showers and freshly laundered clothes. Tim's an idealist, and I'm afraid my shallow values might disappoint him. Looking around, my eyes feast on a hundred shades of green – the olive grey of eucalyptus trees, the jungle green of palms and the mint green of the abundant lawn surrounding the wooden communal house with its kitchen, dining room and wraparound veranda. Everyone has built their own accommodation, while the communal house is used for meetings and workshops.

'Come on, I'll show you our new home. You're gonna love it,' Tim says.

Arms wrapped around each other, we walk up the hill towards the house Tim has built for us. I can't wait to move into our very own place that we don't have to pay rent for. We've both signed up for the dole so we won't have to do tedious jobs anymore. We arrive at a small wooden platform under a redgum tree, with a sagging old mattress with flannel sheets and lumpy pillows, a mosquito net and a corrugated iron roof to keep the rain out. There's barely enough room to accommodate the two milk crates in which I've stored my clothes and books. Trying to hide my shock about the complete lack of luxury our new home offers, we climb up into our makeshift abode, where we sit cross-legged while Tim packs a cone and we smoke some weed.

'Don't you just love this place?' Tim takes a long pull on the bong; the water gurgles as he grins at me.

'It's amazing,' I lie, not wanting to disappoint Tim.

I try to soothe my anxiety by listening to the noises of nature: cicadas, whip birds and the rustling of a goanna on the leafy forest floor. Mum's voice hisses inside my head. *You're living like a hobo under a tree.* But I quickly decide not to listen to her.

We make love and, stoned, I manage to push my worries to the back of my mind. Tim wraps his long body around me as we laugh about all the jobs I've run away or been sacked from since dropping out of university during the first semester.

I roll over and rest my head on Tim's shoulder. He passes me a cigarette and I breathe in its comfort.

'Do you remember how I stank of fish when I worked at Pyrmont fish markets, even when I scrubbed myself afterwards?' I laugh.

'Yeah, that smell was rank, darling.' Tim strokes my hair and face.

'And then I was a sandwich hand in Glebe where Deb, my boss, said I was lazy and stupid, and I walked out in the middle of making a ham and cheese sandwich?' I pass Tim the cigarette and give him a kiss.

'Good riddance to that old cow.' Tim takes a deep drag of the cigarette.

'The most depressing job was at the Maroubra nursing home. The place smelled of poo and urine and the poor oldies were forgotten and alone.' I look at the corrugated iron roof above me. It ticks as the sun warms it.

'Yeah, I don't know how you did that job,' says Tim. 'I was working at the Valhalla in Glebe then, wasn't I?'

'I loved how you'd sneak me in to see movies for free,' I say, squeezing his hand with a flash of pot-induced hope. In this moment, as I gaze through the mosquito net at the red gums that surround us, I decide that I'm going to embrace my new living conditions.

'I remember cleaning that Vaucluse mansion, where I stole two fluffy white bath towels and got the sack.' I giggle, but shame nags at me.

'Yeah, no more shitty jobs from now on. Hey, what about when my dad tried to get me to do an accounting degree? Can you imagine me in a suit and tie?' Tim laughs as he holds my hand.

We smoke some more weed and as I take a long pull on the bong, I decide to ignore the lumpy mattress and the musty smell of the pillows. I'm going to love my new age life, living in harmony with nature.

§

A few weeks after my arrival, days and nights of heavy storms descend. Our mattress, bedding and clothes become damp and musty. We install blue tarps around the sides of our dwelling, which now feels like a prison cell. As the rain drums on the tin roof and fierce winds shake the flimsy tarpaulin walls, I secretly nurture middle-class dreams. I long for a warm house with proper walls, a kettle, indoor toilet and bathtub – a home large enough to walk around in. While I yearn for a washing machine and clothes dryer, I keep a fake smile on my face for Tim's benefit, because I can't admit that I'm fostering dreams of domestic comforts. Mum's voice cackles in my mind. *Ha! You won't last here, you'll see.*

That night, we lie in bed as the rain hammers down and the wind shakes our small dwelling. I'm reading by the light of the torch when Tim starts touching my breasts and kissing my neck.

'I think I'm coming down with a cold,' I tell him as I move away to the edge of the bed.

Tim continues regardless, now nibbling my ear.

'I really don't feel like having sex, sorry.' My libido has disappeared with the rain.

'Fuck this!' Tim jumps out of bed and steps out into the rain. He's a large man, standing just inches away from me on the outside of the tarpaulin. My body freezes and I hold my breath.

This is the first time I've seen Tim angry. I peep through a crack in the tarpaulin and watch him pick up a heavy tree branch from the forest floor. Terrified he's going to hit me with it, I curl my body into the foetal position, making myself as small as I can. I watch him swing the branch above his head and bring it full force against the trunk of the redgum tree that houses our dwelling. The impact of the heavy blow shakes our fragile home. Tim begins to strike the other trees near us. These beautiful gum trees suffer from Tim's violence, and it's all my fault. If I had sex with him, he wouldn't be attacking the trees that share water and nutrients through their intricate root networks. Certain they are sending one another distress signals, I can almost hear them cry out in pain and empathy.

'You don't love me, just admit it!' Tim shouts.

I pretend I'm not there and cover my ears with my hands, my body curled into a ball on the edge of the bed.

Terrified of this new angry version of Tim, I cry silently. My body is not my own and I don't have permission to say no to sex. Instead, I deserve to be punished for denying Tim access to my body. As I lie in silent terror, Tim continues to shout and attack trees, and a dark seed of poison enters our relationship. I don't love this frightening side of the man I thought was gentle and kind.

§

A few weeks later, Tim and I attend a rebirthing workshop conducted by Aurora, a spiritual teacher from Melbourne. Barefoot, we walk into the community hall, where about thirty women and men sit in a circle on the wooden floor. Aurora reads a passage by the Indian guru Rajneesh, a quote that lands an arrow in my heart: 'If you love a flower, don't pick it up. Because if you pick it up, it dies and it ceases to be what you love. So, if you love a flower, let it be. Love is not about possession. Love is about appreciation.'

During the morning tea break, David – a long-haired, bearded man – and his wife, Sally, wander over to where Tim and I sit on the grass, drinking dandelion tea. David passes me a book by the guru Rajneesh, *My Way, the Way of the White Clouds*. On its cover is a photograph of an Indian man dressed in a white kaftan. He has a long silver beard. This is my first introduction to my future guru – the man I will love and follow across the world for the next eight years. As I hold the book with reverence, Rajneesh's mesmerising eyes seduce me to join him on a brand-new spiritual quest.

'He is a truly wise man,' David smiles. 'Please keep the book. Sally and I are leaving next week to live with Rajneesh in America.'

They both wear the signature orange, purple and red clothes of Rajneesh's disciples, and their faces radiate joy.

That night, I stay up reading by the light of my torch while Tim sleeps beside me. Devouring the book as if I was perishing of thirst, Rajneesh's poetry fills me with a shock of wild love, a *coup de foudre*.

'Look for the mysteries in life. Wherever you look – in the white clouds, in the stars in the night, in the flowers, in a flowing river – wherever you look, look for the mystery. And whenever you find that a mystery is there, meditate on it.'

Yes, I want to be a white cloud or a flowing river, floating away from our miserable abode beneath the gum trees. Instead, I'm trapped, our bed is damp, our clothes are growing mouldy and we're enclosed by plastic walls that feel like a prison. We have no money, no options, and I've fallen out of love with Tim. Since his outpouring of rage, all romance has departed our bed.

As I continue to read the guru's words, the rain stops and the first birds announce dawn while I start to think about painless ways to break up with Tim. I want to go back to Sydney to the Rajneesh meditation centre David and Sally told us about. Participating in Rajneesh's transformative meditation practices will allow me to attain the emotional healing and spiritual freedom I long for.

§

A few days later, Tim and I sit smoking weed on the mint green lawn near the communal house. The sun has returned and Tim is topless, barefoot and wearing his favourite torn pyjama pants. Smiling, he passes me the bong.

'I have to talk to you.' My voice is shaky. 'I want to go back to Sydney to live near the Rajneesh centre. This book has changed me.' I pass it to Tim and put my hand on his shoulder.

I explain to him that I want to get a job in Sydney so I can earn enough money to live with Rajneesh at his ashram in America, just like David and Sally. Feeling guilty, I look away from Tim at the veggie garden.

'But you've only been here for a couple of months. I thought *this* was your dream?' Tim's face contorts with rejection, tears streaming down his face.

'I'm sorry. Living here is harder than I thought.' I bite the inside of my cheek and curl my toes.

'Are you breaking up with me?' Tim's sobs are becoming louder, and I lean in to hug him.

'I guess. I'm sorry.' I continue to bite the inside of my cheek.

'You don't even know anything about that man.' Tim's shoulders shake with his sobs.

I hold his hand and stroke his back. In my mind, I've already left him. I secretly relish the thought that soon I'll be living in a house with walls, an indoor bathroom and a bed with freshly laundered sheets. David and Sally told me about the cheap Rajneesh share houses in Darlinghurst that provide homes for new devotees. Tomorrow, I'll phone the ashram to ask about moving into one of their houses. My heart gallops with secret excitement and relief.

CHAPTER THREE

1981

It's a Thursday afternoon and I've been working at Penthouse for a few months. I carry my bike upstairs, store it in the locker room and take off my Birkenstocks and red dress. Changing into my white uniform and red stilettos, I pop three Valium to ease my anxiety, grateful to the Kings Cross doctor who is so generous with his prescriptions. I go into the lounge room, light an Alpine cigarette and pick up my knitting.

The women are busy painting their nails, smoking and plucking hairs from their chins with tweezers. They drink champagne while they chat about clothes, diets, children and their clients.

'I still can't believe you knit, Zoe. It's so old-fashioned. Mum knits too and so does my Nan, but they're *old!*' Stella laughs.

'You can be our granny-mascot.' Donna giggles.

They don't know that my knitting, along with the pills I've been swallowing at regular intervals, helps calm my nerves, a habit I learned from Mum. Despite my desperation to earn lots of money, I remain scared of each new client, especially men who have bald heads, bright blue eyes or cleft chins. The thought of being alone with a strange man continues to be frightening, despite the red duress alarm in the room. Over time, I learn to suppress my fear by mentally adding up the dollars I'm earning and thinking about my guru. I imagine his soulful eyes as they gaze at me, beckoning me to join him at his ashram in America.

It's late afternoon, just before Penthouse's peak hour. We sit at right angles to each other on the white faux-leather couches and watch *A Country Practice*, which Janice has recorded for us. Spellbound, we chat during the advertisements. Maternal Donna is my favourite since she always looks out for me. She's recently got a divorce from her abusive husband.

'He's in Queensland now with his new wife, the poor woman. Good riddance to that prick!' She takes a deep drag on her Marlboro Gold and laughs her smoker's laugh. She supports her three kids and her mother, who also lives with them and babysits while Donna is at work.

Janice has alabaster skin and long black curls. She's married and can't have children. Her husband thinks she works as a receptionist in a five-star hotel in the city. She has a fetish for whitegoods and busily flicks through a glossy brochure with her long purple nails.

'I'm gonna get the new Westinghouse dishwasher. It's super quiet, and I love the platinum look,' says Janice. She leans over to show me a picture of the dishwasher. I appreciate how freely she spends her money and sense she is secretly damaged, like me. All her money goes on top-end electrical gadgets, handbags, shoes and perfumes.

Bridget is the mother of twin daughters. She's putting them through a posh private girls' school that she believes will give them the best chance at life. She passes around her girls' latest school reports in which they both received the highest marks. Her face is full of pride.

'See how clever my girls are? They'll have a better job than mine,' Bridget smiles.

She's planning that her daughters will go to university and have a bright future as doctors, lawyers or perhaps architects.

'I always wanted to study architecture, but it's too late for me.' Bridget gulps her champagne and hides her face behind the curtain of her long red fringe.

I sense her sadness and don't tell her that I, too, went to a posh private school and got the highest marks. I had every opportunity and yet here I am, a sex worker and university dropout without a degree.

Alice, Grace and Nikki are heroin addicts, who support their drug habits with sex work. They seem to float above worldly concerns, and I long to be as hip, thin and alluring as they are. They are huddled together on one of the sofas, looking chill. They're not riddled with anxiety like me.

'Is it true you have a guru?' Grace asks during an ad break. She smiles at me in her detached way. I envy her slim legs and delicate feet that jiggle lazily up and down.

'Yes, his name is Rajneesh.' I'm pleased to tell the women about my guru.

I pass her my mala, the beaded necklace with the locket containing his photograph that I keep in my bag with my knitting, cigarettes and pills. I always put the mala back on as soon as my shift is over, for protection. I explain that the mala has one hundred and eight sandalwood beads that represent the hundred and eight Hindu deities.

'My guru's enlightened, and he lives in America. I'm saving up to live there for a whole year. He's helping me find inner peace,' I say, feeling proud.

My hope is to become enlightened just like him. I believe that if I continue to do his meditations, all my painful childhood memories will be erased.

The women pass around the necklace and peer at his face.

'He's not exactly handsome,' Donna laughs.

'He looks creepy. Are you sure he's legit?' Bridget's eyes are sceptical as she draws keenly on her cigarette.

'Yes, he's the real deal. I'll bring in a video tape tomorrow.' I'm hurt Bridget thinks my guru is creepy.

Mum's voice cackles in my mind. *Look at you, prostituting yourself for a sleazy Indian man.*

I decide not to listen to Mum, and as Bridget passes me back my necklace, I gently hold it, allowing it to give me the strength I need to continue doing my job.

'Zoe, there's someone here to see you!' Paul calls out.

'I'm coming!' I quickly put the mala back in my bag.

Reapplying my lipstick, I check my face in the compact mirror and spray some mint freshener into my mouth to get rid of the cigarette smell.

In the waiting room, Alistair is sitting on the sofa and I breathe a sigh of relief. He's kind-hearted and never wants anything kinky, although his long penis always hurts my cervix. With a bright, lip-sticked smile, I sit on his lap and kiss him on both cheeks.

'This is for you, honey,' Alistair says as he hands me a box of Belgian chocolate and a red rose wrapped in clear plastic with a gold ribbon.

'How did you know I love Belgian chocolate? Let's eat it right now,' I laugh and greedily tear open the wrapping.

'I got it in the David Jones food hall,' Alistair replies as I stuff chocolate into my hungry mouth.

After his shower, I give him a blow job and calculate I've already made six hundred dollars this week. Tomorrow, I'm going to buy the purple satin maxi dress I saw in the window of the House of Merivale, and I'll deposit the rest into my account. Even though I'm desperate to get to America as soon as possible, I'm often waylaid by the lure of clothes, jewellery and hairdos, just like Janice. The new dress will set my trip back by a week, but I convince myself it's worth it.

§

Not all my clients are pleasant. One night, I have an encounter with Gary, a large man with beery breath. He burps and slurs during our faltering conversation as we walk upstairs and enter my room. When the door clicks shut, pure panic grips my stomach.

'Have a shower, Gary, and then we can play.' I try to appear confident.

As I watch him get undressed, I smell his sour sweat from across the room. His eyes have a mean glint. His stomach is enormous, and his body is covered with a thick pelt of black hair.

After his shower, he pushes me to the floor onto my hands and knees and starts to have rough sex with me. I haven't had a chance to apply lube, and I'm too scared to ask him to use a condom. I look down at the grey carpet and tell myself it will soon be over.

'You prissy little bitch, you think you're too good for me!' he slurs.

Each thrust is like a knife. I want to activate the duress alarm, but it's out of reach. I'm trapped, frozen in terror.

He gets off me and sits on the edge of the bed, his legs spread wide, his feet planted on the floor.

'Suck my dick,' he commands.

As I kneel obediently on the floor in front of him, he roughly pushes my head down.

'Open your mouth wider,' he demands.

He is huge as he pushes himself all the way to the back of my throat. Horrified, I gag and submissively bend over him, as my tears drip onto his hairy thighs.

When he has finally finished, I spit into a towel and race downstairs to scrub my teeth, tongue and cheeks with my tooth-brush. I rinse repeatedly and gargle with mouthwash. I open my locker and quickly swallow three five-milligram tablets of Valium and then stand under the hot shower to scour Gary's filth off me.

The water washes away my tears, but I'm still sobbing when I step out of the shower, a towel around me. Donna hugs me.

'Some of them are pricks. Don't let them get to you, sweetheart,' she says.

I lean into her embrace and cry. 'He didn't use a condom and I was so scared. I think I caught a disease.'

Donna tells Paul to ban Gary in future, and I'm grateful I won't have to see him again.

'I'll organise an STD check for you in a few days. And here is a pregnancy test you can use in a week or two.' Paul hands me a small box and places his hand on my shoulder. While I appreciate his kindness, I'm profoundly shaken.

After Gary leaves, I sit on the white couch, my body aching. Gary's taste lingers in my mouth and I chain-smoke my menthol cigarettes to rid myself of his filth. Mum's voice starts in my head. *What do you expect? You're a prostitute, after all.*

But I don't listen to her. What would she know? Everyone is busy with clients, and I'm alone in the lounge room. Soon the Valium kicks in, and I begin to feel a gentle soothing of my heart. I think about weight loss and decide that, from now on, I'm going to smoke and drink coffee all day, and eat only one small meal in the evenings. I'll drop weight quickly on my new diet, and soon I'll be as skinny as the women I work with. My thoughts about dieting provide me with comfort and a sense of control. In my Valium haze, I reassure myself that most clients are okay.

That night in bed, I worry about the effect my job is having on me, but since I have no other skills, working at Penthouse is the only way I'll get to America in a few short months. Each client brings me closer to my guru, who is waiting for me. His promises guide me to him and to his community of devotees.

'A commune is a gathering of seekers, of lovers, of friends, of creative people in all dimensions of life. We can produce a paradise here, on earth,' my guru whispers to me.

The lure of my life with Rajneesh is both consoling and intoxicating, allowing me to lock away my memories of Gary and my childhood secrets. By pushing painful memories to the back of my mind, I manage to keep earning the money I need to be with my guru.

CHAPTER FOUR

1981

On a sun-filled afternoon, Ashika and I lie side by side on our stomachs on my futon. The French doors are open, and warm sunshine dances bright reflections on our faces as we pore over our Herbalife folder, a system of protein powders, weight loss tea and pills that will help us on our quest to be skinny.

'Let's stick to eight hundred calories a day. With Herbalife, we won't even feel hungry,' Ashika says. She lights two cigarettes and passes one to me. I take a deep drag as I hear my blood beat a hopeful rhythm inside my ears.

Ashika lives across the road and we've quickly become close friends since we're the same age and both work nights as sex workers. She has light blue eyes, perfectly placed freckles and red curls that nearly go down to her waist. Our diet goals promise us the perfect bodies to make the money we need to move to America.

Ashika's birth name is Debbie, and she grew up on the Central Coast, one hour north of Sydney. She works at A Touch of Class, a brothel in Surry Hills. We received our new spiritual names on the same day in a small ceremony at the ashram in Darlinghurst.

Ashika pulls up her top and takes my hand. 'Go on, feel how hard my stomach is.'

I reach over and touch her stomach. 'Wow, check out those abs! I reckon I've lost weight too. My jeans are falling off me,' I giggle.

I take the tape measure out of my bedside drawer. We measure our bust, waist and hips, recording the results in our little black book, where we also enter every calorie that passes our lips. I get the scales out of the cupboard and we weigh ourselves.

'I've lost a whole kilo in a week!' Grinning, I jump up and down on the futon.

'I've only lost eight hundred grams,' Ashika complains, her mouth downturned.

'Eight hundred grams is virtually a kilo. You look like total perfection!' I stroke her curls.

We decide to listen to our favourite cassette tape of our guru to inspire us on our spiritual quest.

'I am here to seduce you into a love of life, to help you become a little more poetic, to help you die to the mundane and to the ordinary, so that the extraordinary explodes in your life,' Rajneesh announces.

Ashika taps my shoulder and I pause the tape.

'Our life in America will be amazing.' She grins.

I nod and quash my worries about the weekly donations I've been sending to help fund the American ashram, and the small fortune I've been spending on Herbalife. I decide not to think about my secret spending sprees on clothes and jewellery, or my monthly visits to the expensive Double Bay hairdresser.

'A guy called Joseph has been coming in once a week,' I tell Ashika.

I explain that he's a friendly Jewish man with sad eyes, who asked me to find a girlfriend to visit him at his home with me.

'He wants a girl-on-girl service. He'll pay us three hundred dollars each. What do you reckon?' I ask.

There is a small stab of trepidation about meeting a client outside of work, without the safety of the duress alarm. This is also a sackable offence at Penthouse, but I quickly bury my misgivings with thoughts of the extra money we'll be making.

I tell Ashika he wants us to go over twice a week while his wife is in Brisbane taking care of their daughter's new baby.

'We can make nearly two thousand dollars in three weeks. He just wants to watch us make out, and after that, we'll give him a massage and a hand job. It's easy,' I tell her while stroking her hair.

'Let's do it,' Ashika grins, lighting another cigarette.

§

A few days later, we prepare for our visit to Joseph. Ashika puts on a red mini dress, and I wear my purple satin halter-neck dress that shows off my boobs. We pluck our eyebrows, apply a curling wand and mascara to our eyelashes, draw wings on the outer corners of our eyes using liquid eyeliner and put on foundation and lipstick.

'You look three hundred bucks,' I say, giggling.

Mum's voice inside my head berates me. *You look like a slut!* But I quickly push her words outside of my awareness.

A taxi takes us over the Harbour Bridge to Joseph's mansion located on the waterfront in Mosman.

'Hello, gorgeous ladies.' Joseph greets us with a wide grin, wearing a designer tracksuit. 'Come with me.'

We follow him into the sun-filled kitchen and take a seat at a round mahogany table overlooking the harbour. Joseph feeds us his wife's homemade cherry strudel and challah, a soft sweet bread that reminds me of my Swiss childhood. He picks up a piece of strudel and pops it into my mouth. He passes me a photo of a baby and tells us his daughter has just given birth to her fifth child.

'He's a beautiful big boy.' Joseph looks proud. His eyes have temporarily lost their sadness.

His arms are crossed over his large stomach, his legs spread wide as he watches us eat heartily – an exception for us – but worth every cent we'll earn today. I'm determined not to have any dinner tonight to compensate for the treats. I quickly shove second helpings into my mouth as sugar and fat flood my bloodstream. The gates of my hunger are now wide open and I'm insatiable. Any guilt over deceiving Joseph's wife – who lovingly baked the treats we're now devouring without her knowledge – is swiftly brushed aside by thoughts of the money we're earning.

'Eat up, you're too skinny!' Joseph takes a piece of challah from the cake platter and puts it in Ashika's mouth.

Once we've eaten our fill, he takes us into the living room. We undress and lie on a soft rug in front of the fireplace, where a fire is roaring. The room is cosy with two large velvet sofas, Persian rugs, bookshelves stacked with hundreds of books and expensive artworks displayed on the walls. I'd rather look at the books than take part in a sex performance.

Soon, Ashika and I kiss and caress each other's breasts while Joseph watches us intently, touching himself. I go down on Ashika, and it feels natural to deepen our friendship in this way.

Later, I crawl over to Joseph and give him a hand job while he groans with pleasure. Adept at transforming myself into sexy performative Zoe, my real self carefully hides herself away.

Later, Joseph rolls onto his stomach while Ashika and I tickle his sore back, legs and feet. As we attend to his needs, he tells us stories about his childhood. He spent his early years in Auschwitz until he was rescued by the Americans in the spring of 1945 and migrated to Australia as a refugee.

'Look at this tattoo. It reminds me every day how lucky I am.' He rolls over onto his back and holds out his left arm, sighing deeply.

Ashika and I carefully examine the numbered tattoo until he pulls away and crosses his arms once again, protecting himself from the pain of the past. A rush of empathy overwhelms me.

'I lost my whole family to the gas chambers and came here all alone as a boy.' His hooded brown eyes are once again heavy with sadness. 'Look at this big ugly scar on my stomach.'

He tells us a Jewish doctor had to take out his appendix with a hot spoon, and that he nearly died that day. There were no surgical instruments or anaesthesia at Auschwitz. He screamed and the doctor stuffed a cloth in his mouth so he wouldn't get punished. Joseph's right foot is tapping out a fast rhythm of distress as he tells us his story.

Lightly stroking his scar, tears fill my eyes. His need to be massaged and gently tickled makes sense to me, given the suffering he endured in childhood.

'Roll over, Joseph, and we'll massage your back some more,' Ashika says.

I rub baby oil into his neck and back that are stiff with traumatic memories. Ashika tickles his feet while he groans with pleasure. He tells us how much he loves Australia, where he got to study at university and build a successful accounting business.

'I met my beautiful wife, Hannah, here and we have three daughters and seven grandchildren.' His right foot is still once again.

'I'm so sorry you had to suffer so terribly in childhood,' I tell him as I wipe a tear from my cheek.

§

After a couple of hours, Joseph hands each of us six crisp fifty-dollar bills, leaving us feeling giddy. We catch a cab over the harbour bridge and congratulate ourselves on the easy money we just made.

'Let's check out flights at the travel agent,' I suggest.

Outside the Student Travel office on Oxford Street, we jump out of the taxi and pore over the advertisements in the window.

'Look, there's a return flight to Portland via LA for two thousand dollars,' Ashika says.

'We'll be there in six weeks!' I jump up and down with my hands in the air, right there on the footpath of busy Oxford Street.

'Let's buy our tickets next week.' Ashika hugs me and kisses my cheek loudly.

'We'll also have to pay the monthly five hundred dollars for the ashram's work program,' I remind her.

I calculate that living with our guru for a year will cost six thousand dollars, plus two thousand for flights and one thousand for our spending money.

CHAPTER FIVE

1981

At five-thirty on a Sunday morning, I ride my pushbike up the hill to Satprakash, the ashram on Oxford Street near Taylor Square. The streets are quiet and wet from rainfall, the sky still dark. Having finished my shift at two in the morning, I've managed to get only a couple of hours' sleep, but I never miss the daily six o'clock Dynamic Meditation and the blissful state it leaves me in.

When I arrive, I lock my bike outside and enter the large three-storey building where about forty devotees live together. Hundreds of other disciples live in share houses scattered throughout the surrounding areas of Surry Hills, Paddington, Bronte and Bondi. I live with seven others, half a kilometre from the ashram on Barcom Avenue in Darlinghurst.

Taking off my shoes, I leave them on the rack beside the front door and make my way downstairs to the darkened group room, ready to begin the one-hour meditation that our guru guarantees will bring inner transformation.

Rajneesh declares that the Dynamic Meditation is 'the jewel in the crown' of the many meditations he's developed for his western disciples, and I have complete faith in the healing power of this meditation. Dynamic Meditation is a scientific method to integrate and heal the three parts of the self – the body, mind and heart. The meditation consists of five stages, offering a fast-paced, intense and immersive path to experiencing deep bliss. Designed to last an hour, the practice promises to awaken the meditator's inner awareness, purifying body, heart and mind. Dynamic Meditation provides a way to enter a state of bliss, liberating the body and mind, increasing awareness and activating the authentic self.

Apart from the light of a large white candle, the room is dark. There are about forty of us gathered in the large basement. Since we'll be sweating profusely and throwing our bodies around the room, we strip down to our orange, red and purple underwear. Rajneesh encourages us to embrace our bodies and our sexuality without shame, so clothes aren't a requirement. Ensuring I have a private experience, I put on an eye mask.

Soon, we begin the first stage of the meditation, which involves frenzied music that lasts ten minutes as we perform a chaotic fire-breathing technique. Together, we hyperventilate and dance wildly. Our guru claims that this stage frees the reptilian brain, allowing us to release the control of the prefrontal cortex and become truly liberated.

Desperate to break free from the bonds of the past and from my strict Swiss upbringing, I fully immerse myself in the meditation. With devotion, I put my entire effort into the chaotic breathing that will surely set me free.

The next stage begins, called 'catharsis', and lasts ten minutes. This stage promises to liberate our mammalian brain by freeing old memories and traumas and cleansing blocked emotions. Knowing I have a lot of bad memories to cleanse, I throw myself into this part of the meditation, which involves screaming, crying, shouting and punching pillows that have been strategically placed on the floor.

I love this stage of the meditation because I have permission to have a loud and wholehearted tantrum, which I was never allowed to have in childhood. Instead, I had to be a quiet and obedient child for my parents.

'No, no, no!' I scream.

The next phase is the jumping phase. We jump up and down on the spot and call out 'Hoo, hoo, hoo,' activating our base chakra located at the bottom of the spine. *I'm losing weight as well as meditating*, I marvel. Weight loss is the secret bonus of this part of the meditation because it's an arduous cardio workout. My calves soon burn, and my heart beats hard inside my chest with my intense exertions.

During the fourth stage, we stand in complete silence. Sweat drips down our bodies, which shake from our labours. Feeling high from my exertions, my mind is soaring, entirely free. There is no fear, no anger or worry and I'm open and receptive. Rajneesh teaches that it is in this moment that the busy-minded Western devotee can fully receive the stillness of meditation. Elated, I imagine that my body is being lifted into the embrace of this being who is more than a man. He will save me from myself and from all the childhood pain I've shared with no one.

During the final stage of the meditation, we dance to gentle flute music, our eye masks removed. My arms twirl above my head as I whirl and smile. Every time I participate in this meditation, I become whole. I choose not to think about the way I'm earning money, nor the secrets of the past.

After the meditation, as the sun rises outside, about fifty of us go upstairs and sit cross-legged on pillows placed on the floor of the large meeting room. We watch a video recording of our guru's lecture. It's a time for us to be together, like churchgoers on a Sunday. Taking a seat on the floor next to my friend Sujata, I give her a long hug, close my eyes and focus on my breathing. Happiness courses through my body as I enjoy the sense of belonging to my new spiritual family, a benevolent father figure uniting us.

'Life begins where fear ends,' our guru announces through the large screen.

As I focus on the melody of his voice, I vow to live fearlessly, to discover my highest spiritual self. I gaze at his gentle face and dark, liquid eyes.

'Sadness gives depth. Happiness gives height. Sadness gives roots. Happiness gives branches. Happiness is like a tree going into the sky, and sadness is like the roots going down into the womb of the earth. Both are needed, and the higher a tree grows, the deeper it goes, simultaneously. That's its balance.'

He's speaking directly to me, and I'm captivated by his poetry. Far away from America, yet I am intimately connected to him, despite the distance between us. I want to be a tree that reaches out its branches to the sky, my roots buried deep inside Mother Earth.

'To be creative means to be in love with life. You can be creative only if you love life enough that you want to enhance its beauty, you want to bring a little more music to it, a little more poetry to it, a little more dance to it,' our guru tells us.

Yes, I'm in love with life, and I'm living a life of poetry, meditating daily, listening to his teachings, and making my way through the six hundred books he has published. Rajneesh has a doctorate in philosophy and used to be a lecturer at the University of Jabalpur before becoming a guru. There is so much to learn from this profoundly intelligent man.

Straight after the recorded lecture, Sheela, our guru's private secretary, appears via video link to make an announcement. She is a tiny Indian woman dressed in a purple satin robe, sitting on a bejewelled armchair. Her shiny black hair is cut short, and her large brown eyes sparkle.

'Our beloved guru has told me he has said everything worth saying and has therefore decided to go into silence. He is in a new phase of deep inner bliss, and he's withdrawn from all public duties,' Sheela announces, sounding ecstatic.

My feelings of elation have quickly disappeared with Sheela's shocking message. Shattered, I think about how hard I've worked to hear him speak to me. I long to ask for his advice and to have him touch my third eye in his signature blessing. He's offered the gift of loving attention to tens of thousands of his visitors since 1970. Now that I'm finally about to be with him, he's turned his back on me.

Mum's voice hisses, *I told you your guru is a charlatan. Now he's too lazy to even speak to you!* Squeezing my eyes shut, I whimper quietly, a mere mail-order disciple with no way to absorb his spiritual energy. All I have is the mala with his photo around my neck and the small wooden box with one of his toenail clippings, which he sent to me as a special gift.

Watching my fellow devotees as they absorb Sheela's words in silence, many have their eyes closed, their faces revealing their pain. Others hug and sob, while I sit and hold my face in my hands as tears roll down my face.

Sheela tells us everything will remain the same, that our guru asks us to continue to donate generously so we can expand our desert city in Oregon, where two thousand devotees will live together in harmony.

'Please sell your jewellery or your home if you own one. Remember his words,' she tells us. 'Surrender to me, and I will transform you. That is my promise.'

Secretly resentful, I decide to be an obedient disciple and send him twenty per cent of my income, instead of only ten per cent. This will slow down my savings, but I must remain committed to him and to my spiritual family. When I try to understand his silence, I'm reminded of Mum, who used to stop speaking to us too when she was angry or depressed. Maybe he's tired of being a guru.

The next morning, I banish my negative thoughts, determined to make my way to America, despite Rajneesh's silence. I will still benefit by living on the 'Buddhafield' in his holy orbit. In such proximity, I believe I'll reach enlightenment without him even speaking to me.

Putting on a red skirt and purple t-shirt, I catch the bus into town and get off on the corner of Elizabeth and Market Streets. Rushing into David Jones, I talk to a glamorous young woman at the Christian Dior counter. She carefully applies foundation, lipstick and mascara to my face. Soon I find myself staring at my alluring new reflection in the mirror. I hand over my money, convinced that these new purchases will mask all my flaws and help me earn the rest of the money I need.

CHAPTER SIX

1982

It's eight in the morning and Ashika and I have just returned from Dynamic Meditation. We're wearing matching purple velour tracksuits and sitting in bed, drinking our morning Herbalife shake. Ashika takes a glossy brochure from her red patent-leather handbag, advertising a week-long Bioenergetics workshop. I gaze at photographs of beautiful smiling people.

'This will bring us real healing. Let's take a week off work to do the workshop,' Ashika says, passing me the brochure.

Our guru has developed many therapeutic workshops that promise profound healing benefits and inner growth. He uses a unique blend of Eastern mysticism and Western psychology to help his devotees achieve the spiritual healing we long for.

'Bioenergetics is a body-mind therapy developed by the psychoanalyst Doctor Alexander Lowen. It frees the muscular patterns of constriction held in our bodies from childhood and provides freedom from suffering. It assists people in developing a greater sense of aliveness and acceptance of their bodies and emotions, and it offers participants vibrant healing and freedom,' I read in the brochure.

'Wow, it costs five hundred dollars – that's a lot.' I worry.

'Yeah, but it's run by the famous Rajneesh psychologist, Swami Prasad. He's amazing,' Ashika tells me.

I keep studying the brochure that promises transformation. Perhaps I should do the workshop since I continue to be plagued by memories I've vowed never to share with anyone. Perhaps I'll be cured by this workshop.

'Okay, let's do it,' I say, feeling hopeful I'll be transformed.

Outside, the clear blue sky and winter sun confirm I'm making the right decision. Together we walk up to Oxford Street and go into the Commonwealth Bank to withdraw five hundred dollars for the course.

§

The workshop is held at the Masonic Hall on Bondi Road. On the first morning, we cycle there on our pushbikes, our hearts filled with hope of transformation. The weather is wintry, and we pedal hard against strong winds while dark low-lying clouds threaten rain.

Swami Prasad is tall and dark-haired with piercing blue eyes. He is in his mid-thirties and looks like George Michael from the band Wham, and I immediately develop a crush on him.

'He used to be a Lufthansa pilot, and now he's a psychologist,' Ashika whispers as we take a seat on the floor together.

About forty of us, aged between twenty and seventy, form a circle on the hard wooden floor in the large hall. Prasad takes his seat on the podium in a red velvet armchair, gazing down at us from above.

'Bioenergetics will help you open your heart to life and love. Most of you have hardened your hearts in response to various forms of trauma,' Prasad tells us in his upper-class German accent. 'To go through life with a closed heart is like taking an ocean voyage locked in the hold of the ship. The meaning, the adventure, the excitement, and the glory of living are beyond your vision and reach,' he declares.

My heart thumps hopefully, like a dog wagging its tail.

'If we don't breathe deeply, it reduces the life of our body. If we don't move freely, the life of our body is restricted. If we don't feel fully, it narrows the life of our body. And if self-expression is constricted, the life of the body is limited,' Prasad continues.

As I listen to Prasad's words of wisdom, I breathe deeply and repeat my promise to live with an open heart. I vow to heal from my past. As a feeble winter sun appears through the windows of the hall, my entire being longs for transformation.

'The goal of therapy is more than the absence of symptoms – it is feeling alive, getting a taste of pleasure, joy and love, and taking things more easily. It is vibrant health,' Prasad says.

The floor beneath me is hard while Prasad continues to sit on his red velvet throne. I gaze at the men and women who hang on his every word, united by our yearning to be made whole.

After his introduction, Prasad plays 'Endless Love' loudly – a popular tune by Diana Ross and Lionel Richie.

'I want you to dance and get in touch with your spirit of joy,' Prasad yells over the music.

Dancing vigorously with my eyes closed, sweat drips off me. Secretly hoping that Prasad is watching me dance, I peek out of my half-closed eyelids and realise he is looking at Kendra, a magnificently tall young woman dressed in soft-pink mohair. She is much more beautiful than me, and my heart quickly constricts, my mood plummeting. When the song finishes, we take our seats on the floor once again to listen to Prasad's instructions.

'Focus on your relationship to your breath, movement and body posture. Over the coming days, you'll be investigating your deeply held emotions by performing various physical exercises,' he instructs.

These exercises are like difficult yoga poses that we must hold for an interminable time. Each pose has a specific name such as Earth and Sky Energy, Fill Up and Release, and Horse Stance with Breathing Arms. I hold each pose until I nearly collapse from excruciating pain. We stand for five minutes on one leg, our arms at a ninety-degree angle. *This had better work*, I think as I shake and sweat. Even though I've escaped my family and have a guru, I know there's still something very wrong with me.

'Please allow me to find healing,' I whisper silently.

Prasad continues to watch Kendra, never even glancing in my direction.

§

On the third day of the workshop, I'm wearing my mala and an embroidered red dress, my feet bare and icy cold. I should have brought socks.

'I want each man to pair up with one of the women. Sit with your arms and legs wrapped around each other and focus on your breathing,' Prasad instructs us.

An older bald guy with a cleft chin and bushy eyebrows approaches me. Obediently, I do as I'm told. I breathe deeply and try to get in touch with my base chakra at the bottom of my spine.

'This chakra has strong links with our pleasure and pain,' Prasad tells us.

Our arms and legs wrapped around each other, we breathe in unison to Phil Collins' 'In the Air Tonight'. Suddenly I feel the swami's erection against my stomach. Overcome with disgust, I hit him with my fists. I flail, kick and sob while he cowers on the floor in the foetal position, protecting himself from my fury.

'You pervert pig-fuck!' I cry out.

Tears drip down my face and onto my dress, and on the back of my eyelids I clearly see my uncle's cleft chin and my grandfather's bald head and bushy eyebrows. In a panic, I run out of the hall and onto Bondi Road, where I vomit into the gutter. Traffic rushes past as I heave and cry, while people on the footpath give me a wide berth.

Get a grip, I tell myself harshly, as I try hard to release my traumatic memories into the gutter.

Although the workshop is supposed to be therapeutic, Prasad doesn't come out to check whether I'm okay. When I return to the hall, he's busy helping Kendra, who is crying prettily. This is not what I've paid my hard-earned money for. I want to heal, not unleash unspeakable horror. Ashamed, I feel guilty about hitting the swami, who is crying alone on the floor. No one is attending to his pain either.

'I'm sorry I hit you,' I fawn. I gently rub his back in circles and continue to apologise.

Mum's voice hisses at me. *Don't you dare tell anyone about our family's secrets.*

Quickly, I lock my memories away again and toss the key. After all, I need to keep doing sex work to reach my goal.

Some weeks later, after a routine pap smear and STD check, which our boss Paul has organised for us, the sexual health nurse tells me I have CIN 3, the term for early-stage cervical cancer.

A few days later, I sit in Doctor Maxwell's room, a gynaecologist in Camperdown. He looks at me through his half-rim glasses; his thinning hair styled in a comb-over is held precariously in place with hairspray.

'I know you've been a very promiscuous girl.' His voice drips with distaste.

I'm dirty, damaged goods, and I'm convinced I'll die. I gaze down at my nails, bitten to the quick, with my cuticles gnawed and bleeding after a sleepless night.

'You must be one of those young women who don't use protection when they have sex with random men. If you were more responsible, you wouldn't be in this position. I'm booking you in for surgery next week. I'm sure you've had lots of partners. How many?' he reprimands.

Having lost my voice, I sit frozen and look down at Doctor Maxwell's expensive Persian carpet. I wonder what kind of operation I'll be having. Will they cut my vagina? The Bioenergetics workshop didn't bring the healing it promised, and the princely Prasad did nothing to help me. If anything, things are much worse now.

In my ignorance, CIN 3 stands for a 'sin' – and I have sinned. The disease is all my fault; that's what Doctor Maxwell is telling me. I'll need to take time off work, and I'll have to dip into my savings. *Will I ever get to see my guru now that I have cancer,* I wonder.

When I leave Doctor Maxwell's office, my body is trembling. Outside, cars and buses rush past, the people inside them indifferent to my troubles. Dizzy and afraid, I take a seat on a green park bench in a tiny park littered with cigarette butts, empty chip packets, and crushed beer cans. There's no way I can tell Mum about having Sin Three, a disease that, according to Doctor Maxwell, I only have myself to blame for. She already tells me I bring shame on her.

Her voice hisses, *This is your punishment for doing that disgusting job.* Terrified, I decide to tell no one about my illness. This is one more dirty secret I must keep locked away.

The following week, I catch a taxi to the hospital and home again after day surgery. I tell work and my housemates I'm having a heavy period with bad stomach cramps. Humiliation about being dirty silences me, while Mum's voice continues to reverberate inside my head as I lie bleeding in bed. *You only have yourself to blame,* Mum hisses, just like Doctor Maxwell.

Listening to my guru's tapes on a loop, I swallow large quantities of the Panadeine Forte that Doctor Maxwell prescribed. I lie on my futon for three days, changing my pads every hour to deal with the heavy bleeding. Praying to be released from my shame and dirtiness, my stomach cramps painfully after the surgery. I vow to work harder and to be more careful with my spending after I return to work at Penthouse.

§

Four months later, I've finally saved up for a whole year at Rajneeshpuram. My backpack is ready, and in twenty-four hours I'll be on the plane. Feeling elated, I gaze at my ticket. I have one last task to do, so I load up the dirty white Commodore I borrowed from a friend with milk crates of books, records and clothes that I'll store in Mum and Dad's garage. It'll be a chance to say goodbye to them as well. I get in the car, light an Alpine and slip a cassette tape of Van Morrison's *Astral Weeks* into the player. Turning up the volume, I drive away.

My spirit soars as I sing along to Van Morrison about being born again. Driving past the Pyrmont Fish Markets where I worked for a few months, I remember the smell of fish that lingered on my body and hands despite carefully scrubbing myself. And I hurtle away from all the other jobs I failed at – waitress, masseuse, cleaner, nursing assistant – jobs I had either tried and hated or been fired from. Away from my time at Penthouse – the job that allowed me to save enough money to move to America. I drive past Sydney University where I'd dropped out in my first semester because I felt so stupid and always scared. In two days, I'll be with my guru, free from societal expectations.

Driving through my parents' genteel neighbourhood, I park outside their tidy house and take in the carefully tended blooms in their thriving garden. Mum and Dad meet me at the front door, stony-faced. They look at me disapprovingly through their large matching grey-framed glasses. Mum's face is closed like a fist, her brown eyes cold with disapproval. With her hands on her hips, she steps towards me and sniffs my clothes and hair. She looks at me accusingly and hisses in Swiss German, 'You stink of cigarettes. You'll die of lung cancer at a young age. And why are you wearing those awful orange clothes, and that photo of the ugly long-haired man? I'm ashamed of you, Martina.' A bit of her spit lands on my face.

'You must think carefully about your future, Martina. We worry about the choices you're making.' Dad looks at me with troubled eyes as he crosses his arms.

My hands shake and I look with glazed eyes at the lush garden outside the sliding glass doors.

I want to say to them, *I'm not Martina. My name is Pragito, Song of Love. And I never want a life as uptight as yours. Don't tell me you're happy.*

Instead, with tears stinging my eyes, I mumble, 'I'm sorry I can't be who you want me to be. Please don't be angry!' They still have the power to humiliate me. 'I'm just going to the bathroom.'

In the bathroom, I silently open Mum's red medicine cabinet, where I survey her large supply of pills, which she takes to help calm her nerves. Seresta, Mogadon, Valium, Panadeine Forte, Mersyndol, Rohypnol. I steal a sheet of five-milligram Valium and quickly pop three of them into my mouth. Three has become my magic number since working at Penthouse. I wash them down with water from the tap. The smell of Mum's Chanel No 5 lingers in the bathroom.

Later, we sit in the living room and silently drink Earl Grey tea from the silver teapot and white china cups. As I sit on the white sofa facing Mum and Dad, their disapproval is palpable. The black glass coffee table between us is spotless and we place our cups onto coasters decorated with photographs of the Swiss mountains.

I take a sip of tea as the Valium starts to take effect. I wish I had loving parents who could see that I'm doing something important with my life. Surely a life of love and meditation is meaningful.

Mum stirs fake sugar into her cup. Torn between anger and longing for their approval, I despise them, and yet I still want their love.

'I'm meditating every day and I'm being healed,' I say, my voice taking on a pleading tone.

Mum turns away from me and starts to cry, dabbing at her eyes with her white handkerchief. 'Oh, what have I done to deserve this? I feel like killing myself!'

Crossing my legs, I remain silent and outwardly compliant. But I cannot wait to leave this spotlessly clean and unloving house. Soon, I get up and dutifully air-kiss Mum and Dad goodbye three times on their cheeks, the Swiss way. There is no warmth in Swiss kisses, no hugs or body contact.

'Don't come crawling back to us when everything falls apart for you.' Mum scowls as she stands at the front door.

The Valium is working a treat now, and I drive away from my parents without a backward glance. Van Morrison croons about venturing in the slipstream as I pull into the Golden Fleece service station, where I buy hot chips and a mango Weiss bar. The pills have numbed any remaining hurt. Sitting on the bonnet of the Commodore, I devour my treats and decide not to think about the calories I'm consuming. This time tomorrow, I'll be on a plane to live with my guru.

'And fuck you very much, Mum and Dad!' I whisper and smile.

CHAPTER SEVEN

1983

Standing in line at the immigration desk at Portland airport, I hide my gnawed fingernails from the grim-faced official inspecting my passport. His face and hair are red, and he's built like a tank.

'What's the purpose of your visit to America?' His voice is stern.

'I'm going to work as an au pair for my cousin, to help with her new baby,' I reply, my armpits sweating.

I'm hungover and my mouth tastes bitter from the free champagne I drank on the plane. I'm wearing neat blue pants and a matching cardigan, and have practised my story carefully.

'What are her contact details?' he asks grimly.

I hand him a piece of paper with the details of a Rajneesh devotee who lives in Portland. Giving the official the eye contact of an innocent, I pick at my cuticles. I know the government doesn't want to allow devotees of Rajneesh into America because they mistrust our guru and his red-clad followers. The officer stamps my passport, and I rush outside to look for the bus that will take me to the desert ashram I've dreamed about for so long.

Finally, I spot an old yellow school bus at the back of the car park. About seventy devotees swarm around the bus driver. They wear the signature colours of the sunrise and their mala beads with the locket of Rajneesh's serene face.

Making my way to the back of the bus, I change into my favourite pink dress. Reaching for my mala that is hidden in my backpack, I feel instantly safe as I place the sandalwood beads around my neck. Grateful to be back amongst Rajneesh's devotees, I listen as they chatter in German, French, Italian and Japanese. Taking a seat, the young woman across the aisle smiles at me.

'Hi, I'm Shiva. I'm from Warsaw,' she says in a heavy accent.

'I'm Pragito from Sydney. I can't believe I'm finally here. How long are you staying for? I'll be here for a whole year.' I smile at Shiva.

'Three weeks, my annual holiday from work,' Shiva replies.

'How did you hear about Rajneesh in Poland?' I ask.

'A friend lent me one of his books, and I fell in love instantly.' Shiva smiles.

'Me too. Someone gave me his book *My Way, the Way of the White Clouds*, and that was it. I've been working for over a year to get here,' I explain.

'I'm going to try to do the same next year. It will be hard because our pay in Poland is not very good. I'm a tutor in sociology at the University of Warsaw,' Shiva explains.

'You'll find a way, Shiva.' I squeeze her hand.

§

I doze during the four-hour journey until Shiva touches my shoulder to wake me up. We pass a large wooden sign reading 'Welcome to Rajneeshpuram'. Here is the 64,000-acre ashram and I've finally made it. I reach across the aisle and squeeze Shiva's hand. We smile at each other, her eyes bright with tears.

Once on the property, we drive past a large man-made lake, where naked devotees are frolicking and sunbaking. Ripples of sunshine reflect on the clear turquoise water. We drive past acres of vegetable gardens and thousands of tree seedlings that have been planted since our guru's arrival from India.

We make our way past small townships of prefabricated houses and trailer homes. Tonight, I'll be sleeping in my very own home, finally one of the two thousand devotees living together in harmony. The bus pulls into the town centre's carpark. I gaze at the wooden buildings that look like chalets reminiscent of my Swiss childhood, at a fancy hotel, far too expensive for me, a restaurant, a small hospital, a dental clinic, an ice cream shop, a pizza parlour, a hairdresser, a nightclub and a casino. The bus stops in front of a building marked with a 'Reception' sign adorned by a pair of doves.

Sick with nerves and jetlag, I line up at the registration desk. At last, it's my turn for a handsome blue-eyed French swami – a male devotee – to check my visa and passport then assign me accommodation and a job.

'You must pay five hundred dollars a month for the work program, the Rajneesh Humanity Trust. We need three months up front,' he tells me.

I write out a cheque for fifteen hundred dollars and pass it to him.

The exchange rate is terrible, and I'm concerned about how long my money will last. I'll have to be careful and stay away from the shops.

'You'll be working on the pipe crew, starting tomorrow morning at seven,' he says.

I'm not sure what he means by 'pipe crew', but I'm too shy to ask.

'Your accommodation is at Walt Whitman Grove,' he tells me, then briskly turns away.

Madhu, a bushy-bearded friendly Italian swami in his forties, drives me up a steep hill in his dirty white ute. With my backpack in the tray and the windows rolled down, we drive past a forest of pine trees, their scent fresh and welcoming. After a five-minute drive, Madhu stops in front of a tiny wooden A-frame named Shanti, meaning peace. I already love my new home.

'This is you,' Madhu announces as he proudly opens the door to my new home. Inside, there are three single mattresses on the floor, with only a foot's length between them. At the head of each mattress sits a small pinewood cupboard, where our belongings are to be stored.

'The middle bed is yours.' Madhu smiles broadly.

Stunned by the cramped space, I'm overwhelmed with a sudden rush of panic. I've worked tirelessly to get to my paradise – only to find it's a claustrophobic hut I must share with two others. This is not what I'd imagined. Shocked, I look at Madhu and wonder whether I should catch the next bus out.

'You'll have a great time here,' he says kindly. He pats my back, gets in his ute and drives away.

§

That evening, I meet my two roommates. Krishna is a bearded French-Canadian swami who smells of sweat and takes up almost the entire space. He's tall and must duck his head in the tiny room with its slanted walls. Aisha is a gentle, diminutive Japanese woman in her fifties. She's already lying inside her sleeping bag, looking like a doll.

'I have a job on the pipe crew. What does that mean?' I ask them.

'You'll be digging ditches to lay irrigation pipes. We are growing ninety acres of vegetables here and have planted twenty thousand trees that need water,' Krishna informs me.

My mindset quickly plummets towards despair. I'm paying all my hard-earned money to dig ditches in the desert.

'We work seven days a week, from seven in the morning to seven at night,' Krishna says, full of self-importance.

He explains that work is called 'worship' because the guru says it is an act of love and our way of surrendering to him.

'I work in the boutique where we sell the clothes and jewellery we make here.' Aisha smiles warmly at me. 'Perhaps you will work your way up to a better job.'

'I'm a baker, and I love it.' Krishna puffs up his chest.

He snores throughout the night. To survive, I leave my Walkman and headphones on and listen to Rajneesh's lectures on a loop.

At six in the morning, exhausted, I walk down to the shower block which is filled with naked bodies that chatter in many different languages. Everyone is thin and beautiful. Overwhelmed, I want to run. I hate it here already, and it's not even been twenty-four hours. Then I remember that today I'll meet my guru face to face. He'll do his famous daily drive-by at lunchtime in one of his ninety-three Rolls-Royces. I can't wait to lay my eyes upon him, to be fully seen by him, if only through the windscreen of his car.

CHAPTER EIGHT

1983

At seven o'clock, I report for worship. A yellow school bus picks up our crew of twenty from the canteen and drives us to the site where the vegetable gardens and tree seedlings are cared for. The weather is balmy as we drive through the desert landscape with its hues of brown, red and orange dotted with freshly planted green trees.

A young woman from Brazil with a large thermos sits down next to me.

'Hi, I'm Sujan. You're gonna love our crew. We have heaps of fun turning the desert into an oasis.' She smiles warmly and offers me a cup of chai. It smells delicious, of honey, cardamom and cinnamon.

When we get off the bus, Pema, the German crew leader, gives me a hug. Her black hair is short and spiky, and her bare arms are muscly. She's wearing red overalls, a purple singlet and orange gumboots.

'Welcome, Pragito, we really need more hands on our crew.' Her warm smile creases her sunburnt face.

Pema explains that this is a very important job because we help feed two thousand people every day of the year.

'Here, let me show you what to do.' She hands me gloves, a pickaxe and a trenching shovel.

I begin to use my pickaxe to dig the trench she's assigned me, outlined by yellow spray paint. Once I've loosened the earth, I shovel out the dirt, carefully copying everything Pema is doing in the trench beside me. I'm sweating and dizzy after only five minutes. This is hard labour; how can this possibly be worship?

After an hour of digging, I show Pema the result of my exertion.

'You have to get your trench completely smooth,' she says kindly. 'You'll have to redo this part. See how it's still uneven?'

My heart thumps painfully, my breathing is laboured and my hands have grown blisters despite the gloves I'm wearing. My back and neck are a hot, tight knot. Finally, after hours of digging, my small trench is ready.

'Good job! I know it's hard at first, but you'll soon get stronger,' Pema says, smiling.

She shows me how to lay out the irrigation pipes beside the trench and cut them with a saw. Next, I must smooth the edges with sandpaper, apply purple primer and adhesive, and join them together. I'd rather be a sexy waitress at the Rajneesh nightclub, or a cleaner in my guru's luxury villa. Despite paying six thousand dollars a year to take part in the work program, we're not allowed to participate in meditation sessions or therapeutic groups, so I have lost the very practices that first drew me to my guru. I want to be the best at digging ditches, but my arms and back hurt so much that I start to cry silent tears inside my trench.

Ha! Look at you digging in the dirt and paying all your money to do so! Mum cackles inside my head.

§

After lunch, we line up on the side of the road for 'drive-by,' when our guru takes one of his Rolls-Royces for a spin, gracing us with his holy presence. Two thousand devotees stand along the dirt road and wait for him. I wash my dusty hands and face, apply pink lip gloss and put on my favourite purple feather earrings, feeling pretty and a little sexy. Excited to see my guru's welcoming smile, I wonder whether I've already lost some weight from this morning's manual labour.

Here he is, coming slowly towards me in a powder-blue Rolls-Royce. His companion, Vivek, sits serenely in the passenger seat, an exquisite Englishwoman who has been his most favoured lover and caretaker since she was eighteen. I don't question that he is old enough to be her grandfather. She has a delicate face, straight brown hair and a fringe; the gentle loveliness of a rose. Intense envy stabs my heart.

As the Rolls-Royce draws closer, devotees dance, sing, play musical instruments and wave their arms in the air. Soon, his car stops right in front of me, the electric window rolling down smoothly. He smiles, his eyes hidden behind large Ray-Ban sunglasses. I'm breathless, believing he recognises and loves me. My heart makes an enormous leap upwards, like a fish jumping out of the ocean. But, with horror, I realise he's looking at the petite curly-haired woman standing next to me. He reaches inside the car and offers her a red rose, just like Alistair did with me at Penthouse. She's making ecstatic noises as the two gaze intensely at one another, while he doesn't even give me the tiniest glance.

After a few minutes, he raises the window and slowly drives away, waving his manicured, bejewelled hand. My humiliation is complete, while my fortunate neighbour cries blissfully. Her friends hug her as I turn away, tears of rejection streaming down my face. I hope everyone thinks I'm crying with happiness.

§

Over the coming months, I develop the pipe crew's swagger. I'm proud of my muddy boots, dirt-stained purple King Gee overalls and the honest work I do. My body becomes stronger, and my biceps develop muscle definition. Gone are the days of wearing a g-string and patent-leather stilettos. I belong here in this utopian city, as my friends and I dig ditches, laugh, smoke and drink cups of sweet chai from our thermoses. I love being part of this spiritual family who have travelled here from all over the world to be with our guru.

One overcast morning, my friends Abba, Nabir and I sit inside one of our ditches and blow smoke rings. Workers are given a free packet of cigarettes and two schooners of beer each day. My non-smoking friends give me their cigarettes, so I usually smoke forty menthol Salems a day.

'Watch out! The Mamas coming!' Abba calls out.

Soon we see a fancy black car driven by one of the boss ladies, known as 'Mamas'. They belong to Sheela's gang and their job is to supervise everything that happens at the ashram. Sheela, our guru's spokesperson and private secretary, is a harsh task master, so we quickly put out our cigarettes and start digging again.

§

That night, I lie in the dark amid the snores and farts of my roommate Krishna and think about the money we must pay to live here. Longing for a day off work, I allow myself to question Rajneesh's greed for diamond-studded Rolex watches, Cartier bracelets and Rolls-Royces. A tiny secret seed begins to take root inside my heart as my guru continues to ignore me at his daily drive-by.

A few weeks later, I wash my hands, face and armpits to get rid of the smell of my sweat. I put on my special earrings and brush the dirt off my boots and overalls. I have every intention of going to the drive-by. But instead of lining up along the road, I run up the hill to my little house in the pine forest. Elated, I breathe in the scent of the pines and soon arrive at my tiny home, where I take off my boots and overalls and lie down on the mattress to read quietly in my t-shirt and undies. The pleasure I experience in this moment is exquisite. As I lie on the mattress, I close my eyes and drift into a contented slumber. Later, I water the maidenhair fern that sits on my pine cupboard. Taking a long shower in the empty shower block, I experience a delightful and intimate sense of privacy. We never get a chance to be alone here. Hearing the drums and musical instruments as our guru drives past his devotees, I sit on the veranda of the A-frame, smoke a cigarette and write in my journal, feeling a budding sense of independence away from the clamour of the ashram.

'Fuck you, you never look at me,' I mutter.

Today marks my first small, but significant, act of dissent.

CHAPTER NINE

1984

My guru continues to ignore me, so I seek out the attention of men instead. Monogamy is discouraged by Rajneesh, so 'love' at the ashram is a lot like visiting a lolly shop.

'Free love is your true purpose,' he always advises his devotees. 'The moment love becomes attached, love becomes a relationship. The moment love becomes demanding, it is a prison. It has destroyed your freedom. You become encaged.'

I quickly come to depend on the male gaze as the perfect antidote to my guru's indifference. As one of the youngest women at the ashram, I have some currency here.

One night at the nightclub with my girlfriends, we drink triple-strength Long Island iced teas, smoke Salems and check out the swamis.

'Wow, Vinod is so hot. He's looking at you, Pragito,' one of my friends from the pipe crew shouts over the loud music.

Vinod is from Uruguay, with long dark hair and large brown eyes fringed by thick curled eyelashes. We've been flirting at the cafeteria for the last few days. When he approaches me, we hug and our bodies vibrate with sexual energy. The power of being desired is as potent as a drug that fills the emptiness inside me. We kiss, long and deliciously, bumping and grinding to 'Slow Hand' by the Pointer Sisters.

'You're so gorgeous. I love your energy,' Vinod whispers in my ear.

Feeling beautiful, my heart fills with his craving for me. We dance, the mirrored disco ball, our bodies and my head spinning in unison. As Lionel Richie's 'All Night Long' plays, we sway gently and hold each other close. Over Vinod's shoulder, my girlfriends wave and wink at me from their table beside the dance floor. Between songs, I go over to hug them and gulp more of my Long Island iced tea.

'I love you so much,' I tell my girlfriends drunkenly.

When 'Jump for Love' by the Pointer Sisters comes on, I pull them up by their hands and we dance together in a circle of joy, laughing and jumping. Vinod watches me, the sensation of being desired and the alcohol making my body soar.

When the nightclub closes, Vinod and I catch the bus back to his place. I sit on his lap and we kiss greedily. The bus is bumpy and noisy with laughter and stops every few minutes, dropping off late-night stragglers. At Vinod's house, we rip at each other's clothes and fall into bed. He is a permanent resident here and enjoys the privilege of having his own room.

The sex is impersonal, barely mediocre. He comes quickly, rolls off me, then turns away and falls asleep. I had expected something amazing after the buildup of the flirting at the nightclub. Instead, the sex is merely bland. As soon as Vinod's breathing becomes even, I sneak out of his room. Feeling empty, I walk home and think I must be a bad lover. The next day, Vinod pretends he doesn't know me. He is not the first nor the last to ghost me while I live at Rajneeshpuram.

§

'Immature people falling in love destroy each other's freedom, create a bondage, make a prison,' our guru advised us in one of his past lectures.

Not wanting to be imprisoned, I continue to play the ashram's game of love, juggling two or three men at a time. Soon, I meet an Irish swami called Gopa. He drives one of the big excavators, and as I work with my pickaxe and trenching shovel, we gaze at each other longingly. One day, we have a smoke together. He touches my forehead, gently moving the hair out of my eyes. When our knees make contact, a shock of electricity runs through my body.

The next day, Gopa invites me to his room in one of the townhouses where the permanent residents live, close to our guru's gated home. In his bedroom, he kisses my forehead and cheeks and undresses me, carefully folding my clothes and placing them on a chair. He showers me, washes and combs conditioner through my hair. I'm hypnotised, fully immersed in the experience of being tenderly cared for, the way I never was in childhood. He dries my body, blow dries my hair, massages moisturiser into my skin and carries me to his bed. He touches me slowly, from my head to my toes.

Later, as we make love, he whispers in his lilting Irish, 'I fucking worship you and I want you all to myself.'

This is not what our guru has advised, but Gopa's words are intoxicating, and I'm instantly hooked.

Some weeks later, I wake in the middle of the night. Gopa is on top of me, penetrating me roughly. It hurts, and he bites down hard on my right breast. He holds my hands above my head with one hand and chokes me with his other. I want to push him off me, but I freeze and pretend to be asleep instead. Later, I lie awake and wonder whether this is rape, and what advice my guru would give me, if only he cared.

In the beginning, Gopa provides the gentleness I crave, a holy and sacred feeling. How wonderful his gentle attention feels, as if I were a beloved child. He provides the tenderness Mum never offered me. I go back to Gopa again and again despite the hidden violence. I become the perfect victim, dependent on him while he gradually takes away my power. He pinches my thighs, leaving bruises. He twists my nipples. He chokes me and bites my breasts. Ashamed, I return to him, seemingly of my own free will. Mum hisses harshly, *You have a sickness.* I am dirty and worthless, just like how my grandfather and uncle made me feel when I was still a child.

CHAPTER TEN

September 1984

At seven o'clock in the evening, our crew are eating dinner together in the Magdalena cafeteria on a cool autumn evening. Grateful the long workday is done, I take in the voices of about three hundred people laughing, drinking schooners of beer and eating vegetarian lasagne at long dining tables.

Over the loudspeaker, an announcement advises us of a public meeting in the Rajneesh Mandir, the ashram's large meditation hall. I look at my friend Prakash with a mixture of hope and alarm. Over the past months, seeds of doubt have steadily mounted about my guru and his ashram, which isn't at all like the paradise he promised his devotees. We must pay money to work seven days a week, and don't have permission to attend the daily meditations and therapy groups that first attracted us to Rajneesh. 'Worship' takes precedence. Our guru no longer talks to us so we're deprived of the deep bond we had with him.

Every month, Sheela devises new rules we must obey, resulting in my quietly mounting sense of inner disillusionment. Longer work hours have recently been instated, as well as a rule that we must not own more than twelve items of clothing. Any extra clothes must be given to the clothing pool. Sheela calls this Zen living; apparently our guru wants to free us from our attachment to worldly possessions. Once again, I must force myself to create an obedient, false self, just as I did when I lived with Mum.

'I wonder what's happened?' Prakash asks, her face worried.

For a moment, I wonder whether she shares my secret doubts, but I know not to talk about them.

We put our plates and cutlery into the dirty dish trays and get on one of the buses waiting at the front of the cafeteria. In our work clothes, we arrive at the hall and leave our boots among the hundreds of pairs lined up neatly on racks outside the large glass doors. We find a spot in the middle of the hall as the setting sun breaks through the clouds, casting a magnificent glow through the floor-to-ceiling windows. *This beauty might be a special omen*, I think hopefully. There's a sense of excitement in the air. Prakash and I sit cross-legged beside each other.

'Do you think he'll start speaking to us again?' I ask her.

'Wouldn't that be amazing?' She squeezes my hand.

Since our guru hasn't spoken publicly for three years, our greatest desire is to hear his honey-toned voice in real time. We continue to sit and wait together holding hands, both smiling with anticipation.

Soon, Sheela arrives on the podium. She's sporting a shiny new pixie haircut, a purple silk shirt and a pink velour skirt that matches her expensive rose quartz mala. Despite the petiteness of our guru's private secretary, her power and presence are formidable. She gets to have a private audience with him every day, and as I think about this, my chest and stomach contract with envy.

She takes the microphone.

'Beloveds, I have some very exciting news. Our guru wants to help the most disadvantaged in society – the homeless, addicted and mentally ill – so we are creating a special new program called "Share-A-Home". Soon, we'll be welcoming three thousand homeless people from the streets of America to share the love and abundance we are blessed with at our ashram.'

She explains excitedly that we'll build new A-frames and shower blocks, put up tents and extend the cafeteria. She tells us to sign up after the meeting if we want to be involved in the project.

Since I've always had empathy for those who are rejected by society, I am thrilled and put my name down to work in the Hassid Cafeteria, where I'll be cooking and serving meals and schooners of beer to our visitors.

A few days later, I stand at the reception centre to welcome the arrival of many busloads of mostly homeless men. Looking exhausted, our visitors descend from the yellow school buses, their clothes torn and their stomachs hungry. They are offered clean clothes, a hot shower, medical assessment, food and a safe bed to sleep in. I think back to when I arrived a year ago and how scared I felt.

Smiling, I stand at one of the long trestle tables and hand out clean red, pink and purple jumpers, pants, jackets, socks and underwear. I'm acutely aware of my privilege, having always had a house to live in, enough food in my belly and warm clothes. This is why it's important for me to be of service.

Later that afternoon, I serve up bowls of lentil soup, rice and salad, and for dessert, apple crumble with ice cream, a sense of purpose filling my heart. After dinner, we go outside and sit on wooden benches at the back of the cafeteria to smoke and drink beer, our faces lit by the late afternoon sun.

§

Within a few weeks, however, cracks appear in our new Share-A-Home scheme. Fights become daily occurrences. While standing at the bus stop on my way to work one morning, a brawl breaks out across the road between three young skinheads and two African American guys. Terrified, I watch as they punch and attack each other. When one of the skinheads waves a knife, I run for help, too scared to intervene on my own.

Soon many of the long-term residents have their watches, jewellery and clothes stolen from their rooms since there are no locks on our houses. This leads to resentment towards the visitors, many of live with a mental illness and substance use disorders. Our guru and Sheela clearly hadn't considered this. Another meeting is called, where Sheela angrily shouts in her distinctive Indian English from the podium.

'Three years we have no crime in community. Then new friends come. Now there is fighting and stealing. This is shameful. I bring new friends to our home from the street, and you try to make our home a street. I try to show the world that the ones they call criminals can live beautifully with no crimes, and you bring shame on me with your fighting and stealing. Now I tell you to stand and come up if you're so big and tough. Admit what you did. Show how tough you are,' she yells into the microphone.

A large white guy in his forties stands up, makes his way to the front of the hall and takes the microphone.

'I found this trinket over on the road. By the drive-by. It was just layin' there. It didn't look like anybody really wanted it.' He smiles awkwardly.

'Things don't just lay around in this community. They belong to people.' Sheela's voice is stern.

'Well, I brought it over here, and I had to go to the restroom, so I put it on the table right over there. But when I come out, it was gone,' he mumbles, looking at his feet.

'Just say you took the thing. You stole it. Say that,' Sheela tells him.

'Maybe I did steal it. It didn't seem so though.' His face has turned red.

'Okay. This is your warning. No more stealing. You can go over there.' Sheela summons one of the Mamas. 'Talk to him about returning the thing.'

Filled with sadness, I understand why our new friends are stealing what's always been denied them, including nice watches, shoes and jewellery. They live in a world that has deprived them of their basic human rights, including housing, food and education, and paid work. I think guiltily that I too have been a thief who stole money from Mum's wallet and Dad's trouser pockets.

§

A few weeks later, my friend Leela and I are smoking together at the bus stop on our way to work.

'The Share-A-Home scheme is a ruse cooked up by our guru and Sheela. They only got the homeless people to move here because they're American citizens, which means they can vote in the local elections.' Leela looks grim.

Leela explains that we don't have enough American citizens living here to win an election because most residents come from Europe, Australia, Japan and South America. Shocked at the way we've been lied to, I never even considered that the Share-A-Home scheme might be a scam. How naïve I've been.

That evening, over a drink at the nightclub, Sharma, one of the nurses at the hospital, quietly tells me, 'I'm told to put the drug Haldol in their beer kegs to keep them under control. It's criminal what we're doing to them.' Her face looks stricken.

'Does that mean when I pour their beer, I'm poisoning them?' I ask, shaken and guilty.

Sharma nods, her face serious.

'Isn't that a crime?' I'm gutted that we are poisoning our visitors.

Crack by tiny crack, I'm becoming disillusioned with life at the ashram, which is more prison than paradise. *You're a fool!* Mum's voice berates me. But I'm not yet ready to admit she might be right.

§

It's no surprise that once the local elections are over, our guests no longer have any value. My friend Kohan is one of the bus drivers forced to load them onto buses in the dead of night, only to discard them on the streets of Portland and Seattle, homeless, cold and hungry once again.

'I had to throw them off the bus and take their warm jackets off them,' Kohan tells me, crying.

I put my arms around him, feeling numb with disbelief.

After they leave, I miss them and feel a terrible sense of guilt and shame. By now, there are a thousand tiny cracks in our paradise and my disappointment continues to silently fester. I loathe the authoritarian rules we must obey, Rajneesh's ninety-three Rolls-Royces and having to work seven days a week without a day off.

However, I'm dependent on my guru and spiritual family, and I can't imagine a life without them. Trapped as if in a bad marriage, I'm too scared to leave. Life on my own is terrifying and I'll never survive as an ordinary person in the real world. I can't go back to Mum and Dad, who will surely gloat, and I've lost any friends I had prior to becoming a devotee. If I leave, I'll have nothing to hold on to – no home, no job, no money and, most of all, no sense of belonging.

CHAPTER ELEVEN

1985

One cold evening, we attend another meeting in the Rajneesh Mandir. Sheela stands on the podium dressed in a long, purple satin gown looking like a priestess, her rose quartz mala resembling a crucifix necklace. Her face wears an angry frown, and my stomach flutters with dread. My biggest fear is that I'll be kicked out of the ashram, since Sheela has regularly been forcing dissenters to leave with nothing but the clothes on their backs. I'm terrified I'll be next – that I'll be rejected and abandoned by the guru and spiritual family I depend on.

About five hundred of us sit cross-legged on the faux marble floor. Through the large floor-to-ceiling windows, I watch as night descends and a sliver of moon hangs low in the sky. The hall is cold. I take my friend Shiva's hand and hold it tight. She has one of the most important jobs here, as one of Rajneesh's fine jewellers.

Soon, Sheela begins to shout into the microphone.

'There has been too much negativity at the ashram. This must stop immediately. Our guru is becoming frailer every day because of your negativity. This morning, he told me he will soon die if you continue with your destructiveness.' Sheela's anger is terrifying.

My face grows hot because I have constant negative thoughts about Rajneesh, who's been ignoring me for over a year. I condemn his addiction to luxury goods, bejewelled hats and fancy silk dresses with wide shoulder pads that make him look ridiculous. I fell in love with him when he wore a plain white cotton tunic without any jewellery, and when he owned only one car. Now he's like Imelda Marcos with her three thousand pairs of shoes.

'Our beloved guru's body is so delicate that he will die from your negativity and gossip. It will be your fault if he leaves his frail body and dies, perhaps any day now. This morning, he told me that you are all lazy and must work harder to create his vision of our perfect paradise,' Sheela shouts.

We're already working twelve hours a day. What more does he want? I think, biting the inside of my cheek. I'm scared of Sheela, just as I was of Mum, and any sense of freedom and joy has evaporated.

'I don't want to hear any complaining or gossiping from anyone. I have spies everywhere. They observe everything you do and say, and our beloved guru demands complete obedience. Nothing less will do, or he will die. If you're not in agreement, you can leave right now. Go on, stand up and get out,' Sheela yells.

No one moves. I look at the floor, feeling a complex mix of guilt and resentment. When the meeting is over, we shuffle out of the hall in silence, avoiding eye contact. As I tie the laces of my boots, Shiva whispers, 'I hate this,' her face hidden behind her long dark hair.

'Sheela's a bitch. Now we're not even allowed free speech or to think for ourselves.' My heart is dark and heavy.

'I've never told anyone, but when he wants a new piece of jewellery, we have to do twenty-four-hour shifts. If we don't finish in time, he has a tantrum like a three-year-old.' Shiva cries softly.

'I can't believe it,' I say. But I can.

Shiva weeps with exhaustion, having just completed a long stint crafting a new diamond ring for him.

'How much jewellery does he need?' she hisses.

He's like a bowerbird collecting shiny things, I think bitterly as I put my arms around her.

§

We, his devotees, are paying for his insatiable greed by doing sex work and by gifting him our life savings and our parents' inheritances. The more we give, the more he wants. *If only I had the courage to leave him*, I think. But I'm dependent on him and on his devotees, who have become my family, and I know I'd be lost on my own. Hugging Shiva, I wipe the tears from her cheeks, grateful we can share our secret thoughts.

'Come stay at my place. I don't want to be alone tonight,' she says.

'I'd love that,' I reply as we walk arm in arm in the dark towards her trailer.

I suck on a cigarette and dig in my pocket for my last two Panadeine Forte. I chew and swallow them without water while Shiva and I hold each other tightly, grateful for our friendship and shared secrets.

'I wonder where the peace has gone?' I whisper as we sit on Shiva's bed in her pyjamas, drinking ginger tea.

We turn out the light and, as I try to go to sleep, I admit to myself that I'm starting to hate living here. I'm sick of digging ditches. I can't stand sleeping with two other people in a claustrophobic room. But what will I do and where will I go if I leave?

§

A few weeks later, at breakfast, the pipe crew are sitting outside the cafeteria in the sunshine. I'm drinking black coffee and taking deep drags on my cigarette while the pipe crew eat their banana porridge. I'm dieting, so a cigarette and hot drink will do.

There's an announcement over the loudspeakers. 'Make your way to Rajneesh Mandir.'

I put out my cigarette, get on one of the buses waiting in front of the cafeteria and take a seat at the back.

'I wonder what Sheela wants now. Twenty-four-hour shifts?' I grimly ask my friend Prakash from the pipe crew.

Soon, we make our way in our stockinged feet to the middle of the hall. Terrified, I wonder whether our guru has died because there's been too much negativity. I am still unable to control my bad thoughts, and I'm worried people can see the negativity emanating from my head like thick black smoke. For the next sixty minutes, we sit and wait on the cold floor. Whispers travel around the hall.

Suddenly, there is a collective gasp as a silver Rolls-Royce pulls up at the back entrance to the hall. The room becomes perfectly silent. Our guru exits the car and glides onto the podium wearing white socks and thongs, a shiny black silk robe with wide shoulder pads and a hat adorned with jewels. He looks unsteady on his feet, and I'm worried about his fragile health. Sheela was right; *he will* die soon. But how will we go on without him? He takes a seat on his bejewelled armchair. My heart pounds in my ears.

After three years of silence, our guru speaks. Tears stream down our faces as we listen to his melodious voice.

'My dear friends. Sheela and her gang have fled the ashram with fifty-five million dollars belonging to me. Sheela has betrayed me.' His voice is stern.

An outcry reverberates through the hall while a shockwave travels through my body.

'Sheela and her gang have committed countless crimes,' Rajneesh continues. 'She has attempted to murder my physician, Devaraj, by lethal injection.'

A roar of anger erupts, while my stomach knots with anxiety.

'Sheela carried out wiretapping throughout the ashram, including recording me in my private rooms. She poisoned three thousand homeless people with tranquilisers, and she planned to murder the people closest to me. I had no knowledge of any of her crimes until yesterday,' Rajneesh announces.

The hall is filled with shocked silence.

'Sheela is a fascist dictator. I promise you that things will be much better now that she has gone,' he continues.

I weep with relief and hope, convinced that everything will improve now that Sheela is gone and the guru I've loved for three years is speaking to us again.

§

In the weeks that follow, Rajneesh returns to giving daily lectures, often speaking to his devotees for a full two hours. We work less and enjoy a newfound freedom without Sheela's strict surveillance.

One day after lunch, Shiva and I share a cigarette. 'Rajneesh is a smart guy. There's no way he didn't know about Sheela's crimes. I don't trust anything he says.'

'Do you really think so?' I pass her the cigarette, feeling numb.

Over time, the pipe crew become lazier, our work ethic slipping. I turn up late to work, and we spend afternoons smoking and gossiping near the ditches we're meant to dig, trying to make sense of the sudden changes that have occurred at the ashram. Most believe Rajneesh was unaware of Sheela's crimes, since he was 'in silence' during her four-year reign. Still, a hidden part of me suspects he was aware of – and may have even orchestrated – the crimes and deceptions carried out by Sheela and her gang of women.

That afternoon, our guru addresses his devotees, his voice laced with deep hurt.

'I allowed her total power because I believed in her devotion and her love. But power corrupts.'

§

As I catch the bus to the Magdalena cafeteria one morning, I watch with astonishment as a large convoy of black government cars arrive. At breakfast, word quickly spreads that the FBI are here to investigate the crimes Sheela has committed over the past four years. They spend days interviewing the residents, uncovering widespread wiretapping and large stockpiles of Haldol used to subdue our homeless friends and other defiant devotees.

My friend Leela, who's been working as one of the ashram's nurses, is interviewed by the FBI.

'I had to confess I put Haldol in the beer kegs to keep the homeless people sedated. I might get arrested,' she says guiltily.

'Every phone call and every conversation in our bedrooms has been recorded – we've been under constant surveillance,' Prakash tells me that afternoon while we're digging a trench.

'This isn't the paradise we were promised,' I reply grimly.

My fingers are sore from nail biting. Feeling violated and numb with shock, I don't know how to make sense of the revelations of crime and corruption at the ashram.

Although our guru has resumed his daily lectures, I continue to doubt his claims that he was unaware of Sheela's crimes. On one hand, I experience feelings of euphoria that Sheela has gone and our guru is speaking to us again. On the other, I mistrust Rajneesh's declarations of innocence.

'She has betrayed me. She has betrayed my people. She has betrayed the commune. My whole trust was shattered. They managed to keep me almost like a prisoner under the pretext of protecting me,' he declares one morning.

Is he a victim or is he complicit? I wonder over and over.

When the last of the pills I brought from Australia run out, over a year later, I find myself drinking large quantities of alcohol every afternoon after work, desperate to silence the heartache I can no longer hold back.

§

Some weeks later, on a sun-filled autumn day, as I walk to the cafeteria for lunch I watch a Lear jet take off into the clear blue desert skies. I don't know yet that our guru is on board, together with his personal physician, Devaraj, and his long-time companion, Vivek. When we find out he has abandoned us without a goodbye, we are as bereft as orphans. Soon, Rajneesh is arrested and deported, banned from ever returning to America, leaving two thousand devotees forsaken and adrift.

Grief-stricken, I stop working on the pipe crew, sleep in and cycle rapidly between feelings of loss and freedom. I return to doing my morning and evening meditations, praying for guidance towards the next right step. Every day, hundreds of devotees leave the ashram on yellow buses. Most must beg for travel money, relying on the kindness of their families and friends.

'My dad is sending me money to return to Germany. I'll have to move back in with my parents, because I don't have money to rent even a small room,' Leela tells me over a beer.

After weeks of feeling immobilised, I ring Mum and ask her to send me money for a flight home.

'I told you this would happen,' Mum says, sounding smug.

'Thank you for the money, Mum. I don't know what I'd do without you,' I say, feeling shamefaced.

When the funds arrive, I book a flight home to Sydney, knowing I'll miss the many friends I made at the ashram terribly. In Los Angeles, I spend the night in a hotel near the airport that I pay for with Mum's money. I drink spirits from the mini bar and cry myself to sleep. I even find myself missing my roommates – alone for the first time in over a year. The next morning, I board my flight to Sydney.

Within a few short weeks, the ashram is bankrupt and desolate, our utopian dreams shattered. Rajneesh's ninety-three Rolls-Royces are sold and the 64,000-acre property is bought by a Christian organisation and later becomes a youth camp for Christian teenagers. How swiftly everything has unravelled; our beautiful dreams have come to nought.

§

When Rajneesh moves back to his former ashram in India in 1986, I try hard to stay away from him. The glow of devotion has evaporated. Yet life back in Australia makes no sense without the spiritual connection I've depended on for the past five years. I've lost the friendships I made in my teens, and my parents are living back in Switzerland once again. My Rajneesh friends continue to provide my only sense of belonging.

Disillusioned yet unable to stay away, I visit Rajneesh at his Indian ashram three times between 1986 and 1989. In this way, I remain stuck in an unfulfilling, dependent relationship with my indifferent guru, unable to stand on my own two feet.

CHAPTER TWELVE

1987

After Rajneesh returns to his former ashram in Pune, India, my visits to him are each only six weeks long. I still don't know whether Rajneesh knew about Sheela's crimes, or about the authoritarian regime she'd created in America. I suspect that perhaps he'd orchestrated everything together with Sheela. I long for my past devotion to my guru to return, yet I no longer believe in the paradise he promises his devotees during the daily lectures he's resumed in India.

Still, I remain emotionally reliant on him and on the spiritual family I've been part of throughout my twenties. Most of my friends have already gone back to be with him. I envy their unwavering faith, while I've become a half-hearted devotee, secretly consumed by doubt. Yet, I continue to crave my initial feelings of ecstasy when I first fell for him all those years ago. He is my disappointing father, and his cult is my dysfunctional family, and I can let go of neither.

One rainy September morning in 1987, I walk down Oxford Street in Darlinghurst to buy a coffee. I shelter beneath my umbrella and check out the window of the travel agent, where I spot a cheap flight to Mumbai. In that moment I succumb once again to my enduring craving for my guru, who is still my favourite drug. Perhaps he's changed back to his former self, before he became addicted to luxury goods.

In the travel agent's office, my heart beats a fast rhythm of hope as

I resolve to re-devote my life to him. Staying away from him means I am alone and lost. If I offer myself to him wholeheartedly this time, his spiritual sustenance will surely bring about the inner transformation I yearn for. Recommitting myself to him will allow me to receive his divine blessings. Life is empty and meaningless without him, so I must go back to him and try once again to be healed.

§

Three weeks later, I board a plane for India. In Mumbai, I get on a noisy bus reeking of rich spices and body odour. We travel along chaotic roads crowded with cows, wheelchairs, buses, old cars, bicycles, motorbikes and rickshaws, all heading in different directions. Drivers hurtle in no apparent order, beeping their horns in a noisy cacophony. After a four-hour journey, I arrive in Pune, where I climb into a rickshaw that takes me to the ashram. Finally, with sweat trickling down my back and armpits, I arrive in the upper-class suburb of Koregaon Park, where stately mansions are set in large well-tended gardens. Exotic birds call out their songs and monkeys play in the native Tetu and Chandan trees.

When I stand at the gates of the ashram, I cry tears of relief as I take in the sunrise colours of hundreds of devotees. I belong with this spiritual family, and I immediately feel less alone. I can't wait for my guru to transmit his spiritual radiance onto me. Soon, the crowd streams into the gleaming white marble-floored Buddha Hall. My heart beats a rhythm of joy, and my knees and hands shake. Today I'll meet my guru again and this time, things will surely be different.

He arrives on the podium with his companion, Vivek, whom I have loved and envied from the beginning. She's his favourite disciple and has lovingly dedicated herself to his care for fifteen years. She looks serene, still a gentle English rose. I wish I had her calm composure and quickly vow to be more like Vivek, instead of my unruly, disloyal self. I'll meditate every morning and evening and think only positive thoughts.

We bow down to our guru as we sing in unison the ancient Buddhist declaration of devotion.

'*Buddham saranam gacchami.*' I go to the Buddha for refuge.

'*Dhammam saranam gacchami.*' I go to the Dhamma for refuge.

'*Sangham saranam gacchami.*' I go to the Sangha for refuge.

I don't question Rajneesh's portrayal of himself as the Buddha's equal, or the expectation that we kneel and bow down before him as if he were a god. Regressed, childlike and needing rescue, I bow down and worship him. I'm in his care, a small child in the presence of a father-figure.

At the Indian ashram, only those devotees with wealth and beauty are offered the privilege of living with our guru inside the ashram's gates, so I move into a tiny flat, about fifteen minutes' walk from the ashram, in an ugly concrete apartment block that I share with three flatmates. Still under construction, our home is little more than a building site. I have my own room that costs just ten dollars a week. The windows are open to the elements, without any glass, and I sleep on a lumpy futon which I've bought from the previous tenant for fifteen dollars. The flat has only cold water, so my flatmates and I use an electric coil to heat water for bucket showers. I also learn to use a squat toilet. I love everything about India, most of all its joyful, noisy chaos, so different from the tidiness of Australia.

My friends and I rent pushbikes to attend morning and evening meditations as well as Rajneesh's daily lectures. Looking frail and unsteady on his feet at age fifty-six, he graces us with his presence every day in Buddha Hall. I reconnect with old friends from the pipe crew and I fall for Prem, a guy from Brazil with the softest skin and deep brown eyes. I could gaze into them forever. We know each other from when we lived at the ashram in America.

§

When I return to Sydney six weeks later, I'm disappointed that I didn't receive the spiritual salvation I'd hoped for. Once again, I decide to devote my energies to the rescue romantic love might bring. I miss Prem and feel empty and alone without him. We write each other long declarations of love and soon, he follows me to Australia and moves in with me. We're deeply in love, but our intense romance takes an unexpected turn when I start vomiting days and nights.

Prem and I are in the doctor's office when he informs us that my illness is due to me being pregnant. In this very instant, I inexplicably fall out of love with Prem, devastated that my body has betrayed me. Feeling no trace of maternal instinct, I make a swift decision to terminate the life growing inside me. I'll have an abortion and be sterilised at the same time, because the drudgery of motherhood is not for me. I don't want to end up like Mum, depressed, trapped, cooking and cleaning. I don't allow Prem any say in my decision. Within days, I break up with him, as if it's his fault alone that I'm pregnant. My feelings for him have turned mysteriously from romance to revulsion. When Prem moves out, I show no compassion for his feelings of hurt and confusion. I think only about my guru, who's indoctrinated us not to have children.

'A woman cannot become enlightened if she has a child. Children harm a woman's spiritual development – they turn her into a slave. The nuclear family is a disease, one of the greatest traps that society has used for millennia to keep man and woman a slave,' he advises us repeatedly.

I agree with my guru's words. After all, Mum was trapped in a family system that was deeply unhappy. She told us frequently that she was a slave to us and that she wished she had studied medicine instead of becoming a wife and mother.

After many phone calls, I find a gynaecologist in Ashfield who agrees to perform a termination and sterilisation at the same time, even though I'm only twenty-six years old. It will cost a huge sum of money but I don't care how much, because I refuse to be entrapped in the grind of motherhood.

On the day of the surgery, I take a taxi to the private hospital in Ashfield, the chambers of my heart firmly closed. I fill out the forms and sign away my foetus as well as my future fertility. My breath is shallow, my pulse racing. I lie on a gurney in the hallway outside the operating theatre, feeling cold and alone, an anonymous young pregnant woman wearing only a blue hospital gown and a red plastic wristband.

'Beloved guru, you are my guiding light – I'm doing this for you,' I whisper, trying to reassure myself that I am making the right decision. On the gurney, my stomach contracts with fear.

After the operation, I wake up crying in the recovery room, a light-blue waffle weave blanket wrapped tightly around me. A nurse strokes my forehead as I sob and try to tell her the world is a frightening place. I have no control over my weeping or the dark thoughts that have invaded my brain.

'You've had a bad reaction to the anaesthetic,' the kind nurse tells me.

She gives me a hot water bottle for the stomach pain, a couple of Valium, a cup of sugary tea, an egg and lettuce sandwich cut into triangles and two shortbread biscuits. I quickly devour the food and medicine while my stomach cramps painfully. I gently touch the two scars on my belly. Bleeding onto a thick pad between my legs, I think of Mum and how she'll finally kill herself if she finds out what I've done. *You stupid, heartless girl!* she hisses.

I tell myself that I'm finally a devoted disciple, now that I've taken this step against the norms of obligatory motherhood. I convince myself I've made the right decision. But there is another smaller voice inside me that whispers I might have made a mistake.

After the surgery, I catch a taxi back to my friend's house where I'll be staying for a few days. Tears stream down my face as I lie in bed. Unsure why I'm crying, I'm gripped by fear and loneliness. I binge for hours on bread with thick hunks of butter smothered in honey, a large tub of Greek yoghurt and a block of chocolate, my comfort foods from childhood. Insatiable, the bingeing continues for days, while my stomach cramps painfully and I bleed bright blood onto the large pads I must change every hour.

CHAPTER THIRTEEN

December 1989

I'm visiting my guru in India for the third time. Riding my bike to the ashram, I pass the chai wallahs selling sweet chai from their mobile carts and park my bike outside the ashram gates. I enter the hall, take a seat among the other devotees and wait for our guru to arrive.

'Vivek died last night in a room at the Blue Diamond Hotel,' my friend Prakash from the pipe crew tells me.

'No! It can't be true.' My eyes fill with tears.

The news of Vivek's death spreads quickly through the crowd.

Last night, my friends and I were partying, drinking Margaritas by the swimming pool of the Blue Diamond Hotel, while she died alone upstairs. I always thought Vivek was the luckiest of all our guru's devotees. I can't understand why she would want to end her life. Overcome with terrible guilt over the way our spiritual family have failed her, I cry silent tears for Vivek.

Soon, Rajneesh arrives in a cream-coloured Rolls-Royce. He enters the hall, sits on his handcrafted throne and says nothing. He doesn't mention Vivek or the profound suffering she must have endured, causing her to commit suicide. Appearing indifferent, he fails to give tribute to her years of loyalty. He doesn't thank her for loving him so well; he doesn't even look sad. Indifferent, he says nothing at all.

I dig my nails into the palms of my hands in silent anger. Vivek died an untimely death, aged only thirty-eight. Her birth name was Christine Wolf Smith. She was born and raised in England and died all alone in a room of a fancy hotel in India on the ninth of December 1989.

In the late 1970s, Rajneesh used to talk tenderly about Vivek.

'I had a girlfriend when I was young. Then she died. But on her deathbed, she promised me she would come back. And she *has* come back. The name of the girlfriend was Shashi. She died in 1947. And now she has come as Vivek to take care of me. Vivek cannot remember it. I used to call Shashi "Gudiya", and I started calling Vivek "Gudiya" also, just to give continuity. Life is a great drama, a great play – it goes on from one life to another to another,' he told his devotees.

I don't understand why he won't talk about her now. As I sit on the marble floor, I can't forgive his silence. His eyes are dark pools of indifference.

When we leave the hall, I run into my friend Shiva. 'Vivek has already been cremated, and we're not allowed to say farewell to her,' she tells me.

'Why not?' I say, dumbfounded.

'There won't be a funeral for her, because suicide is a cowardly act,' Shiva replies.

Distraught, I sit by myself in the smokers' area. My entire being hurts for Vivek, this beautiful, deeply private and dedicated woman. Swallowing a couple of Valium, I take in long breaths from a beedi, a thin Indian cigarette wrapped in tendu leaves. I eavesdrop as devotees nearby discuss her suicide.

'Vivek was spineless,' says a middle-aged, bearded guy with long grey hair.

'She's so selfish, leaving him all alone,' another replies.

I don't hear a word of empathy towards her. She slept in our guru's bed and catered to his needs for fifteen years. I can only imagine the agony she suffered in her final days. We're supposed to be a compassionate family, so we're all responsible for her death.

'I'm so sorry, so very sorry, dear Vivek. We've failed you – each one of us, and most of all the man you loved so well,' I whisper.

This refrain repeats inside my head for hours. I hate my callous guru, and I'm ashamed of the cult I've been reliant on for so many years. As I light another beedi to suck down my anger, I remember reading an interview with Vivek when she first became Rajneesh's devotee, in which she described her deep love for him.

'And then you see that he's full of life. And he's glowing, just totally glowing, and his face is just auras and auras and auras of gold. He just looks like gold and gold and gold!'

But today, there's no aura of gold. Our guru has finally shown his true colours – those of a petty, self-serving man.

The day after Vivek's death is the day I finally find the courage to break up with my guru for good. I return alone to my room on the building site where I'm suddenly overcome with a high fever. I shiver and shake on my mattress and, as the night stretches on, I let go of my love for my guru. The mistrust I've carried since my time at the ashram in America has finally reached its conclusion, and I know in my bones I'm forever done with him.

'Vivek wanted to go back to England to seek treatment for her depression, but our guru wouldn't let her go,' one of my flatmates tells me.

I hold Rajneesh responsible for Vivek's lonely death. He didn't allow her to get the help she needed to treat her mental illness. The next afternoon, filled with a new resolve, I catch a rickshaw into town and book my flight home. With my ticket in hand, I return to my tiny room and pack my rucksack.

'I'm done with you,' I mutter viciously.

I want to tell my friends that our guru is a fraud and that they too should get out, but I know they won't understand my decision to break free of him. I berate myself for the long years of dependence and Mum joins the refrain inside my head.

You stupid, stupid girl!

I resolve to change my name from Pragito back to Martina, the name I was given by my parents. I whisper it to myself, and it sounds like a beautiful promise: 'Martina'. Rajneesh's indifference about Vivek's suicide is the final straw.

I can't wait to get away from him, to go home to Sydney and rip his pictures off the walls, burn his books and tapes and cut my red, purple and orange clothes to shreds. I'll hurl his stupid mala into the ocean and I'll never wear the colours of the rising sun again. I'll take a hammer and smash the pathetic wooden box with his toenail clippings that I treasured.

'You're dead to me!' I mutter, feeling only hatred.

My rage empowers me to walk away from my years of dependency. I make a vow to follow my inner knowing, even if it takes me a lifetime. With my rucksack on my back, I board the bus to Mumbai, soothed by the pungent aroma, noise and clamour of India. That night, I catch a flight home to Sydney, knowing I'll never again be dependent on a guru, determined to find my own truth.

Tonight, thirty-five years later, I look out at the flashing lights of coal ships entering Newcastle harbour. I light a rose-scented candle for Vivek the English rose – Christine Wolf Smith – who died all alone in a hotel room in India. Bringing my palms together in front of my heart in the gesture of namaste, I honour her divine radiance with the light within me.

'Dear Vivek, may you be at peace and may you rest deeply where there is no sorrow, but only ease, freedom and joy,' I whisper.

CHAPTER FOURTEEN

1989

I wake in Sydney in the early morning. My body tingles with jet lag and a thrilling sense of purpose. Today I'll rid myself of every trace of my false guru. I get out of bed and put on a loose red dress. Soon I'll no longer be wearing red. I rummage through my drawers and find the letter I received from Rajneesh when I became one of his mail-order devotees. I read the name he bestowed on me: 'Ma Prem Pragito, Song of Love'.

Sobbing, I rip up the letter and burn it in the kitchen sink with my lighter. I'm Martina now, not Pragito and certainly not a 'Song of Love'. Full of loathing, I rip the pictures of my former guru off the walls. I tear up his books and use a hammer to smash his cassette tapes and the mala I wore for the past eight years. Next, I take the hammer to the wooden box my guru gave me, containing one of his toenail clippings.

'I don't want your filthy toenails. I've wasted years of my life on you,' I howl.

My boyfriend and I are living on Campbell Parade in Bondi, where our tiny flat looks out at the beach. The weather is stormy, the waves a wall of grey as I run onto the beach with the remnants of my mala and wooden box. I throw them into the waves and cry as I kneel on the sand, praying to be released from the curse of my former dependence on the guru.

'Let me go; let me stand on my own two feet,' I sob.

When I return to the flat, I sit on the floor and get to work shredding my clothes. I attack my favourite soft-pink dress, orange low-cut blouse, red hippie skirt and the purple satin halter-neck dress I'd bought for an outrageous sum at the House of Merivale when I was still a sex worker for my former guru.

'I hate you,' I yell, as I destroy dozens of pieces of clothing and throw them into green garbage bags, together with the shredded books, cassette tapes and posters.

Sweating, I fill eight large garbage bags and drag them to the back of the flats where I dump my former life into the communal bins. I return upstairs and whisper my name over and over – a powerful new mantra.

'Martina, Martina, Martina.'

Freeing myself from my former addiction to the guru, I vow to be fierce and independent.

Later, I catch a bus to Bondi Junction and go into Just Jeans, where a sale is on. I try on a black t-shirt and black jeans and look at myself in the change room mirror. I'm liberated – a woman in black.

'Can I pay for these and leave them on?' I ask the shop assistant, who smiles and cuts off the tags for me.

I buy three black t-shirts and two pairs of black jeans, then I go next door and purchase some Doc Martens.

'I'm done with you,' I mutter as I dump my red clothes into the bin outside the shop.

At the florist, I buy some sunflowers to celebrate my liberation and catch the bus home, feeling elated.

'I'm free,' I whisper as I sit on the bus holding my own hand lovingly.

§

On the nineteenth of January 1990, Rajneesh dies of heart failure, aged fifty-eight. It's rumoured that his physician Devaraj administered a lethal injection because he was tired of his life as a guru. Following Rajneesh's death, the Indian ashram is rebranded 'Osho International Meditation Resort'.

Thirty years later, the resort continues to attract two hundred thousand visitors every year, and his followers still spread their guru's message from numerous Osho Meditation Centres located in cities across the world.

PART TWO:
SEARCHING

CHAPTER ONE

1989

Soon after I leave the guru, I start to have nightmares about my Swiss grandpa and uncle. Horrified, I see Grandpa's wrinkled face, bald head and bushy eyebrows and smell the stench of his putrid breath. I picture Uncle's cleft chin, thick black hair and piercing blue eyes. I catch the scent of tobacco from his wooden pipe and hear him sucking on it. In my nightmares, I'm trapped with these two terrifying men who live in a respectable white terrace house in a genteel neighbourhood of Basel, my hometown in Switzerland.

Feeling like a small child, I'm terrified of my relatives' enormous hands, the hard snakes between their legs and their huge hungry mouths. I'm Little Red Riding Hood, devoured not by one but by two wolves. Their hands hurt me, and their mouths swallow me up. I feel a sharp pain between my legs. These shocking sensations appear like pieces of a jigsaw puzzle, forming a terrifying picture.

One night, I wake from a nightmare, convinced my relatives are in the bedroom of our Bondi flat. They loom above the bed, ready to pounce, while I lie frozen in sweat-soaked sheets. When I finally gather the courage to move, I get up, swallow three Valium and wash them down with a glass of water. Chain-smoking, I sit on the couch and look out at the shadowy waves on the beach, too scared to go back to sleep. I wish I could lock my memories away, but they continue to invade my consciousness. I know they are real, and I can no longer ignore them. Instead, I must pay careful attention to them.

I suddenly realise that my guru and spiritual family allowed me to escape my childhood trauma. The day I became Rajneesh's devotee, I believed I was reborn – a brand-new person, a young woman without a past. Rajneesh even gave me a new name and a new birthday. How cleverly I tried to escape my past. Back then, I loved the name Rajneesh gave me, Pragito. The name Martina came with such sad and heavy burdens.

I gently rock back and forth on the couch, trying to soothe my distress and waiting impatiently for the Valium to take effect. As I light another cigarette from the end of the last, I reflect on how foolish I'd been to believe I had no past and that all my problems disappeared the moment I became Rajneesh's devotee. Now that I'm Martina again, I can no longer escape myself. Walking away from the guru is like falling down a deep, dark hole. Chain smoking, I realise I gave the guru all my power, believing in miracles that never materialised.

I turn on the television and watch *Rage* on the ABC. The song 'Never Tear Us Apart' by INXS is playing. While Michael Hutchens swivels his hips, gorgeous skinny women with large lips and sexy eyes bump and grind beside him. If only I could be one of the beautiful women in the music video. They look so free, while I'm no longer fun or sexy. My boyfriend will break up with me if I don't pull myself together. We haven't been intimate for three weeks. I never want to have sex again, yet years of abuse and sex work have ingrained in me the belief that sex is all I'm good for. As the Valium kicks in, I pray to be released from my memories. Weak and exhausted, I lie on the couch.

'Free me from my pain,' I whisper over and over.

§

My flashbacks worsen over the weeks that follow. Memories of abuse haunt me, even during the day when I'm awake. This is how I find myself in a psychiatrist's office on Ocean Street in Edgecliff. Nauseated, I sit on the worn blue and beige tartan couch in Doctor Goldberg's waiting room, the polyester fabric itchy against my legs, my armpits sweaty.

Soon, the large, red-faced, bearded psychiatrist ushers me into an office filled with dark furniture. The curtains are drawn and the room is gloomy; only the green lamp on his desk sends out some rays of light. Doctor Goldberg takes a seat behind his giant desk, while I cower on one of the hard high-backed chairs in front of him. Too ashamed to tell him about having been in a cult, I can't bring myself to utter the words 'sexual abuse,' because I'm scared he'll judge me. He takes notes on a large yellow notepad as he fires questions at me.

'Does anyone in your family have a mental illness? What do you do for work? Are you sexually active? Are your parents alive? Are they married or divorced?'

I cry as I answer his questions – they seem irrelevant to me – but he continues writing, his eyes focused on his notepad.

What is he writing? Does he think I'm crazy?

Eventually, he passes me a clipboard and instructs me to fill out a questionnaire called the Beck Depression Inventory. I circle the answers to the forty-two questions while tears drip onto the page.

I am sad all the time, I'm utterly worthless as a person, my future is hopeless and it cannot improve, I am a total failure, I would like to kill myself, I have lost interest in sex completely, I feel I'm being punished.

'You're suffering from depression in the extremely severe range,' he tells me after he scores the questionnaire.

I know I should tell Doctor Goldberg about the sexual abuse, but I can't, because he's a man with a university degree, an authority figure like Grandpa and Uncle, while I'm a failure doing menial work. In 1989, childhood sexual abuse isn't yet spoken about.

'This should help you. Take one tablet every morning,' he instructs.

Doctor Goldberg takes out a prescription pad from his desk drawer, writes out a script for Prozac and swiftly dismisses me. The consultation has lasted no more than fifteen minutes.

I walk back out onto Ocean Street, blinded by the sunlight, mascara smeared down my cheeks. Leaving the consultation more distressed than when I arrived, the diagnosis of 'extremely severe depression' makes me feel worthless and doomed. I'm a depressed woman, just like Mum, and I'll end up with a life like hers.

CHAPTER TWO

1990

My friend Trish and I are drinking coffee at a sticky round table at the Tropicana Café next to the Kings Cross fire station. Trish has also recently left our former guru and we've formed a bond over this difficult experience. She works as a psychologist with patients who have an HIV diagnosis. My abuse memories come tumbling out and I whisper them to Trish so no one else can hear. Shame fills my stomach and my body shakes as she holds my hand and looks into my eyes.

'Oh Martina, I'm so sorry,' she says kindly.

She tells me about a psychologist in Bondi Junction who works with survivors of sexual abuse. Trish says I need professional help and that it will take time, but I'll heal.

Later that day, I call the psychologist Trish suggested. While I sob down the phone line, Doctor Miller offers me an appointment the following Monday.

On the day of my appointment, I arrive half an hour early. I sit in the waiting room on the first floor of a seventies brown brick building on the corner of Old South Head and Bondi roads. A Mozart piano sonata plays softly in the background. It does nothing to calm me. Listening to the muffled voices that come from inside the counselling room, I can't make out any words. As I wait to meet Doctor Miller, my legs pump up and down like pistons, and I chew the cuticles of my thumb, ripping off a large strip of skin. Blood drips onto my jeans.

Ashamed, I wrap my thumb in a tissue to stem the blood. I want to run onto the street and home again, to hide under the safety of my doona. Finally, the door to the counselling room opens while I look at the floor – I don't want to have eye contact with the patient leaving the office.

'Come in, Martina. Please call me Robbie,' the psychologist says, shaking my hand.

Robbie is in her mid-forties and has short grey hair. Her body is motherly, with soft folds on her stomach. I feel a small glimmer of hope that she might be able to help me. We sit opposite one another on cream-coloured IKEA armchairs. She is wearing a calf-length denim skirt and low-heeled boots. Her hand-knitted pink cardigan makes me feel safe. Her slow breaths are reassuring, and I yearn to be mothered by her. The counselling room is light-filled, with thriving pot plants on the bookshelf and on the floor.

Soon, my childhood story pours forth like a muddy-brown waterfall after a heavy storm. Robbie leans forward in her chair, nodding as she listens without interrupting me.

'Mum left me at Grandpa and Uncle's house every few weeks. She was depressed and needed a break from being a mum.' Tears trickle down my cheeks.

Robbie passes me a box of tissues.

Suddenly, I'm overwhelmed by a full flashback, flooded with a torrent of memories that threaten to bury me.

'I must kiss Grandpa, and he touches me down there – his fingers are like snakes. He has mean eyes, bushy white eyebrows and horrible brown moles on his bald head.' My body shakes as I recount my memories to Robbie, while the morning traffic rushes by on Old South Head Road.

The flashback continues to unfold.

'Uncle also lives with his parents. He's handsome and nice to me and makes me laugh. I love him,' I tell Robbie.

But at nighttime, when everyone is asleep, he comes into my room.

'Uncle is two different people: a charming one, and a monster who hurts me when no one is looking.' I hyperventilate from the terror I feel.

'Martina, I want you to breathe in to the count of four, and out to the count of six. Let's do it together. Breathe deeply and allow your stomach to expand and contract. Put your hand on your belly. Now push your feet into the floor so that you can ground yourself in the present moment. Remind yourself you are an adult living in Australia, and you've survived your Swiss childhood. These three practices will help regulate your emotions. You can practise them any time you need to calm yourself,' Robbie explains, her voice gentle.

I slow my breaths, put my hands on my belly and push my feet into the floor. I tell myself I'm an adult, safe from the reach of my relatives.

'I love Uncle, but I'm so scared of him. When he dumps me after he's hurt me, I know I'm dirty and worthless,' I cry.

I wonder whether Robbie believes me. The memories are so awful they seem far-fetched – even though my body knows I'm telling the truth. But soon I wonder whether my mind has a sickness that makes me imagine things. Maybe I have schizophrenia.

'Do you think I'm a liar?' I ask her.

'Martina, I believe you. Your memories are very detailed. Why on earth would you make them up? If the abuse hadn't occurred, you wouldn't feel so distressed. I'm so sorry you experienced sexual violence by your two relatives. No child should have to suffer as you have,' she says gently.

'Why didn't Mum, Dad or Grandma notice I was being abused?'

I cry tears of relief to finally be able to reveal the secrets I've locked away for two decades.

At the end of my first session, Robbie gives me a diagnosis that feels more accurate than the one Doctor Goldberg gave me.

'From everything you've told me and from the symptoms you describe, you're suffering from complex post-traumatic stress disorder. This refers to violence that occurs over numerous occasions during childhood. You developed this condition because no safe adult was available to stop the sexual abuse from happening, and because there was no one to provide comfort. No one intervened. Instead, they all looked the other way,' she explains.

Sobbing, I listen to her words, a balm to my wounded heart. I love Robbie already. How different she is to Doctor Goldberg, who handed me a script for Prozac and dismissed me as swiftly as he could. He diagnosed me with depression but didn't ask the right questions to discover what lay beneath the depression.

'I'd like to see you for weekly sessions. Is that okay with you? I will give you a reduced rate because you're a victim of crime,' Robbie suggests.

'Yes, please.' I blow my nose into a wad of tissues.

Robbie's diagnosis explains my suffering, and I'm relieved there's a name for my desperate state. My thumb throbs where I ripped off the cuticle in the waiting room. I hear the coo-cooing of a pair of doves outside the window, and am amazed that normal life has continued around me, while my own world has shattered.

From this day forth, Robbie becomes my trusted healing companion. Over the next three years, I attend weekly therapy sessions, during which I experience profound distress but also life-changing healing. Robbie teaches me that I had the misfortune of being born into a family where sexual violence against girls was normalised and where no one cared enough to notice my distress. It's taken more than twenty-five years for me to find the courage to give voice to my secrets. Finally, I've found someone to witness my pain, someone who believes and assures me that I can heal.

CHAPTER THREE

1990

I sit across from Robbie during our weekly therapy session, frightened of the memories I'm about to face. I want to flee onto Old South Head Road and disappear into a world that is free from pain. But there is only one world now – a world full of danger and darkness. In the counselling room, I go back in time to when I was four years old.

'I'm sitting in the backseat of Mum's blue Mini. I feel special being in the car without my brothers,' I tell Robbie.

Mum doesn't tell me where we're going, and I'm too shy to ask because her mood is sombre. We drive through the autumn landscape as the sky darkens. I look up at the trees with their bare branches; a few wrinkled brown leaves still cling on. We're driving away from our village, towards the city of Basel. Tall buildings loom above us while dread builds steadily inside my stomach.

'I'm sick of being everyone's slave,' Mum mutters from the front seat of the car.

In the counselling room, terror spreads and takes over my body. I start to cry.

'Mum is taking me to the scary house,' I sob.

We are in the middle of town now. Green trams ring their bells, and high school students smoke at the tram stop. They laugh together and I want to be carefree, just like them. If I was a teenager, I would stand with them and smoke, free from the fear that continues to build steadily inside me. The streetlights light up, so pretty, but there's no comfort now that I know we are headed to the scary house.

'Mum will leave me there. I want to beg her not to, but I know to keep my mouth shut,' I whimper.

'Remember you're on a different continent. You've survived. Imagine you are sitting on a train. Observe the landscape outside the train window. The landscape is the past, and you're safely on the train in the present time – an adult living in Sydney,' Robbie reminds me.

Mum parks the car outside my grandparents' terrace house. We walk to the front door. Mum carries a bag containing my clothes and pyjamas. I have my own toothbrush at Grandma's because I stay there so often. My body is rigid with an acute sense of danger. Mum rings the doorbell, and Grandma opens the door. She swoops me up in her bosom and calls me her *Liebling*, her sweet darling. I smell her powdery lavender scent and bask in the warmth and affection she provides.

'Mum's dropped me off and has driven away without a backward glance. She doesn't like her parents or her older brother, and she's fed up with being a mother – that's why she leaves me there,' I sob.

'Tell me what's happening now that your mum has left,' Robbie says.

'Grandma takes me into the kitchen. She gives me a glass of milk and some sweet biscuits,' I say.

The kitchen smells of spices, vanilla and sweet honey. Grandma is rolling and shaping potato gnocchi for dinner; her homemade tomato sauce bubbles on the stove. I listen for sounds in the house, but all is quiet. Grandma chats while she drops pieces of gnocchi into the boiling water, and I do some colouring-in at the kitchen table while I drink my milk and eat a sweet biscuit.

I try hard to colour only inside the lines but Grandpa starts shouting from upstairs, and Grandma rushes to attend to him. I stay at the kitchen table. I know I'll have to go upstairs and kiss him later. I hear Grandma fuss over him while I continue my colouring-in, which is outside the lines now because my hands have started to shake. The sweet biscuit suddenly tastes like cardboard in my mouth.

'I'll have to go upstairs to kiss Grandpa,' I tell Robbie, crying.

'Take slow deliberate breaths, push your feet into the ground, and remember you are safely in Australia. Your abusers can't hurt you now, and your grandfather is no longer alive,' Robbie reminds me.

A key turns in the front door and my handsome, twinkling, blue-eyed uncle comes into the kitchen, bringing the cold in with him. He tickles me and makes me laugh, despite myself. He kisses me on my lips and scratches my mouth with his bristly stubble. I try not to look at his scary cleft chin. He always tells me that murderers have cleft chins and I'm very scared he'll kill me.

'Uncle has just come home. I love him, but I'm scared of him,' I tell Robbie. Uncle is funny and charming, but I know he'll turn into a monster at any moment.

'A four-year-old can't make sense of the grooming process. Your uncle deliberately deceived you by making you love him, so that it would be easy to abuse you,' Robbie explains.

'I know Grandma loves me, but she won't protect me from the two bad men she must obey,' I cry.

I'm so scared, with Grandma upstairs and Uncle tickling me, that I wet my pants. Warm wee trickles between my legs onto the wicker chair. When Uncle leaves the kitchen, I take off my wet stockings and mop up the wee under the kitchen chair. Ashamed, I hide my stockings at the bottom of the kitchen bin.

'*Liebling*, go upstairs and give Grandpa a goodnight kiss,' Grandma says to me when she comes back down.

Since his stroke, he spends all his time in bed. In the therapy room, I hyperventilate.

'I'm right here with you, you're not alone,' Robbie says with her soothing voice.

The stairs are steep. I want to beg Grandma to let me stay in the kitchen with her, but I know I must be a good girl. With my short legs and small four-year-old body, I climb upstairs, holding on to the wooden banister. As I reach the top of the stairs, Grandpa's old man smell hits me, with its undertone of stale urine. I enter the room and see the horrible plastic bottle on his bedside table, filled with his dark-yellow urine. I approach the bed to kiss him, as instructed.

'Oh Robbie, I don't want to,' I whimper. 'He smells so bad.'

I hold my breath. His bald head, bushy white eyebrows and mean, grey eyes terrify me.

'He grabs my hand and puts it under the blanket on his snake.' I weep as I recall the memory.

In the bedroom, I dissociate by making myself as light as a balloon. I manage to escape by flying to the corner of the ceiling, where I gaze down at the peppermint tea in the cream-coloured cup sitting on the bedside table next to Grandpa's bottle of urine. From the corner of the ceiling, everything has become unreal, distant and foggy. I'm hardly breathing.

'His fingers are hurting me,' I cry.

'You did nothing to deserve the abuse he inflicted on you. He was a dangerous paedophile,' Robbie reassures me.

§

That night, Grandma bathes me, helps me brush my teeth and tucks me into bed. She reads me *Little Red Riding Hood* and cuddles me. I breathe in her lavender smell. I'm scared of the wolf. She holds my hands as we say our goodnight prayer.

'Dear God, keep our family safe, and thank you for another day of blessings,' she prays.

If only God could keep me safe. The house is silent. As I lie in bed, I hear the door ease open and a small crack of light comes in from the hallway. A large shadow appears and moves silently towards me. Here is the monster I fear most. I pretend to be asleep, but I know he can hear the loud pounding of my heart. He moves closer. He smells of pipe tobacco. His shadow looms above me. I want to call out to Grandma to please help me. But she's in bed with curlers and a hairnet on her head, and earplugs in her ears because of Grandpa's snoring.

Once again, I dissociate and transform myself, becoming as light as a balloon. Dissociation allows me to leave my body and protects me from my terror and pain. In the corner of the ceiling I float near the streetlight that shines into the bedroom. Down on the bed, the monster harms my mouth and throat so I can't breathe. Later, he hurts me between my legs. After a long time, he grunts and disappears, but I don't come back into my body for ages. Awake, I listen for noises.

In the safety of the therapy room, I cry so hard I'm scared I might never stop.

'Martina, put one hand on your belly and the other on your heart. Breathe in and out slowly. You are safe now. Your perpetrators don't have the power to hurt you anymore, and you didn't deserve the abuse they inflicted on you.' Robbie looks at me with the kindest eyes.

'But what if I did deserve it?' I whimper.

'No child deserves to be abused. And remember, they'll never be able to hurt you again,' she reminds me.

Later, Robbie holds a mirror in front of my face and tells me to gaze into it.

'You are a strong young woman. You live in Australia. You are safe, and the abuse took place thousands of miles away.' Her voice is soothing.

My breathing slows as I recognise my face in the mirror. I'm an adult, no longer four years old. I blow my nose and drink from the glass of water Robbie hands me.

'Look at your hands. What do you notice?'

'They are big. They are grown-up hands,' I reply.

'You've worked hard today. Go gently into your day and remember to be a kind friend to yourself,' Robbie says.

CHAPTER FOUR

1990

Robbie is the first person I've revealed my secrets to and, after six months of attending therapy with her, she's become the most important person in my life. It takes courage to go back to her every Monday. As I sit in her calming presence, buttery yellow sunshine streams through the open windows and I hear the distant rumble of the morning traffic on Old South Head Road.

I go back in time to 1968. I'm seven years old and today, Dad will travel to America for three months. He's been chosen to take part in a course for important men at Harvard Business School, where he'll learn to become even better at his job. Dad never stops telling us how successful he is at work.

'Mum and Dad are having a fight just before he leaves for America. I watch them through a crack in the door as they argue. Mum's shouting that he hasn't given her enough money for food,' I tell Robbie.

I listen as Dad tells Mum she can make do with the cans of food and the apples and potatoes from the cellar if she runs out of money. She continues to yell at him while he picks up the paper, avoiding eye contact. Now Dad's ignoring Mum. She hates it when he does that. The more he ignores her, the more she shouts. Doesn't he know that by now?

My hands are squeezed tightly, and I hold my breath. Mum stands over Dad, her bony shoulders hunched in pain and rage, while he sits on the white sofa holding the paper in front of him like a shield. Mum's face is contorted. I can't see Dad's face because it's behind the paper. If I could see him, I think he'd be smiling the false smile he wears when Mum's angry with him. He's wearing his good grey trousers and his best shoes that Mum polished for him last night. She's also ironed his shirt and trousers with perfect creases. His shoes stick out beneath the newspaper, while I crouch on the cold tiled floor of the landing. Dad's large black suitcase is waiting next to the front door, and I wonder whether I might fit inside it.

I don't want to stay with Mum. Dad doesn't yell and he's always nice so he's my favourite parent. He has blond hair and blue eyes, and he walks with bouncy steps, while Mum has grey hair, sad brown eyes and a long, gloomy horse face with a big nose. I never have to fear Dad. He only hits us on our bare bum with the cane carpet beater when Mum tells him to. So it's her fault, not his.

Wouldn't it be wonderful if Dad and I could live together, just the two of us, I daydream. We'd make spaghetti in the evenings and have chocolate ice cream every night. Life would be perfect with just Dad and me.

But Dad walks out the door without me. He can't wait to begin his exciting new life in America without us. He gives me a quick kiss and leaves in a taxi without a backward glance.

'My life is a misery!' Mum yells after he leaves. 'I might as well kill myself!'

She disappears into the bathroom to take some of the medicine that helps calm her nerves.

'You must leave for school in five minutes. Don't forget to brush your teeth,' Mum calls out to my brothers and me.

She slams her bedroom door, and I hear her pull down the grey metal blinds so she can lie in bed in her darkened room. Brushing my teeth, I listen to her sobs and wonder whether she'll be dead by the time my brothers and I get home from school.

§

At school, I worry about Mum all day. I walk home with Marianne and Irene, the sisters who live next door. It's a warm summer afternoon, and I try hard to pretend I'm an ordinary girl with a happy family. In their garden, we pick tiny strawberries and raspberries, warm from the sun. The berries are juicy, with a sweet and slightly sour tang. I climb over the back fence and into our garden, the lawn an immaculate, cheery green.

'Robbie, I don't want to go home after school,' I cry.

My backpack feels heavy and my stomach is full of giant brown moths, their fluttering wings making me ill with dread. I slip off my shoes at the back door and tiptoe into the house, listening with radar ears. I sneak into the bathroom and lower the black toilet lid to stand on the toilet in my socks. Silently, I open Mum's red medicine cabinet and look inside her boxes and bottles of medicine: Valium, Mogadon, Rohypnol, Seresta, Codeine.

Counting Mum's pills, I try to work out which ones she's taken. I try to remember how many there were yesterday and how many are now missing. I'm only seven, but I've already become an expert on Mum's pill use and the likelihood that she might overdose – maybe even right now. Scared of Mum's rage, I'm much more afraid of her long silences after she's taken her pills. Easing open the door to her bedroom, I tiptoe into the darkened room. The grey metal blinds are tightly shut. I take in the dark shape of her body. The room is cold.

Mum is lying on her back under her blue-and-green chequered mohair blanket. She looks like a corpse. Perhaps she's already dead. Holding the fingers of my left hand close to the tip of her nose, I check whether she's breathing. I can feel her faint breath just below her nostrils. I'm relieved we are safe for now.

But immediately, I start worrying that Mum may never wake from her sleep. Perhaps her shallow breath is that of a dying person. I put my hand in front of my own nose to compare Mum's breath with mine. Mine is stronger. What will happen to us if Mum dies, with Dad all the way in America? I think about ringing the police or an ambulance, or I could go next door and ask Marianne and Irene's mum for help. I decide to go back and check Mum's breathing again in a few minutes, and sneak out of the room.

'I was often scared that Mum might be dead when I got home from school,' I tell Robbie, crying.

'Oh Martina, this must have been so painful. You and your brothers were burdened by a mentally-ill mum who was trapped in an unhappy marriage. Her suicide risk was very real. You were the parentified child watching over your mum at just seven years old.' Robbie's validation soothes my heart as I sob into a wad of tissues.

§

It's a Sunday morning in 1973 and my parents are sleeping in. I'm twelve years old and wearing my red pyjamas and blue reindeer slippers. Sneaking into the bathroom, I lower the black toilet lid and stand on it to look through Mum's medicine cabinet. This has become a consistent routine. On the spur of the moment, I steal one of her pills. Today, I won't be Mum's guardian, tasked with preventing her suicide. Instead, I decide to join her in the practice of swallowing pills to ease my own secret feelings of despair. I pop a tiny Valium tablet out of the blister pack, fill the toothbrush glass with water and swallow the small, pale-yellow pill. I return to my room and lie down on the bed to read my book. I begin to feel woozy after about twenty minutes, and gradually my sad heart becomes light and free – such magic from this one tiny tablet. Its tender, delicious buffer amazes me.

Soon I begin to seek out this freedom from pain regularly, swallowing relaxants, sleepers and painkillers. I steal only one or two at a time and keep a small stash of them in my hiding spot – inside a pair of rolled-up winter socks in the back of my wardrobe. I use the pills whenever I need that magic protection – when Mum is angry, when I'm afraid she'll hurt herself or when Mum and Dad are fighting. By now, I've had a five-year apprenticeship observing Mum's pill consumption. Since she doesn't know how to regulate her own emotions, she can't teach me how to regulate mine.

'I can't believe I was stealing Mum's pills when I was twelve,' I say, embarrassed to reveal this secret to Robbie.

I tell Robbie that I still use pills every day to help me cope with my constant despair. I admit to her that I get scripts for Valium and I buy Mersyndol and Panadeine Forte over the counter at the chemist. I always take three tablets at a time, but I don't tell her that because I'm too ashamed.

'This is very understandable, Martina. We learn by watching our mothers, and a child's bond with her mother is her first relationship. Martina, we can work together and reduce your pill use. Would you like that?' Robbie asks gently.

'I would, but I'm really scared to live without them.' I feel deeply embarrassed.

'We can make a plan and do it gradually. I'll support you,' Robbie suggests.

Nodding compliantly, I'm secretly resistant. I'm not ready to face life without the comfort of pills, and I quietly hope Robbie will forget today's conversation and never mention it again.

CHAPTER FIVE

1991

I've been attending weekly therapy with Robbie for eighteen months. Five minutes before the end of our session, I have a sudden brainwave. I laugh and clap my hands.

'Robbie, I'm going to write a letter to Uncle to confront him about the sexual abuse. I want him to admit what he did to me and he'll have to apologise.'

My heart is a galloping horse of hope inside my chest. Confronting Uncle will resolve my constant sense of powerlessness. When he admits his crimes, I'll have the healing I long for. I'm excited and empowered as I imagine his apology.

'Robbie, writing the letter means I'm a brave survivor,' I say excitedly.

I'm sick of being a pathetic victim.

'Maybe we could slow things down a little, Martina. Think about the possible consequences. How will you feel if he denies the abuse? I'm worried you'll be devastated all over again, just as you are starting to feel stronger. Most paedophiles never admit their crimes,' she says carefully.

But I refuse to listen; I'm in full flight, imagining his shame, remorse and apology. I'll finally be vindicated.

'Martina, let's wait until our session next week, so we can talk through the pros and cons a bit more?' Robbie suggests, her brow furrowed with concern.

Instead of taking Robbie's advice, I rush home and compose my letter on thick cream paper using my black fountain pen and my most grown-up handwriting. I will keep the letter short, containing only the facts.

Uncle A

I remember what you did to me at your parents' house in Basel.

You sexually abused me when I was a small child, every time I came to stay with you. The sexual abuse took place on the first floor in the front bedroom, and on the top floor in your bedroom, as well as in the bathroom. You hurt me many times. I was helpless and without protection. Your father, my grandfather, also sexually abused me in the same house.

I want you to admit the crimes you committed against me and to apologise for harming me.

I will send copies of this letter to my mother and father, my brothers and your ex-wife, Alice. They, too, need to know about your crimes.

Martina

I rush down Oxford Street to the Paddington Post Office before it closes. I buy five airmail envelopes and stamps, and ask the tall postmistress in her blue uniform to make four photocopies of the letter. Excited and full of purpose, I address the envelopes.

But as soon as I drop the letters into the red post box, I panic. Terror quickly spikes inside my body, starting in my stomach and chest. My hands tingle and I suddenly feel faint. Uncle will punish me. Why hadn't I considered that? I want to run back into the post office and ask the postmistress to retrieve the letters for me, because

I've made a big mistake. I should have listened to Robbie. I stare at the red letterbox in horror. What have I done?

That night, I dream Uncle is on a plane bound for Australia. He catches a taxi from the airport to my tiny terrace house in Paddington. He's brought a handgun with a silencer attached, just like in movies about the Mafia. He stealthily breaks into my well-locked house and makes his way upstairs into the bedroom, where I lie curled on my side, sleeping. He puts the gun into my mouth and pulls the trigger, muzzling me forever. No one hears the muffled sound of the gun.

I wake covered in sweat, my body shaking. *I shouldn't have posted the letter; I shouldn't have posted the letter; I shouldn't have posted the letter.* This refrain repeats inside my head as I realise I've put myself in grave danger.

For three long weeks, dread loops endlessly, and I check the mail several times each day. Finally, there's an airmail envelope in my letterbox, addressed in Uncle's almost illegible handwriting.

Dear Martina

I am deeply offended at your unfounded accusations. I am your loving godfather and uncle and have always cared for your safety and happiness with tenderness. I have only ever laid the gentlest hand on you.

Your extended family and I know all too well that you have an unfortunate history of being unstable and a liar. Your letter confirms that you belong in a psychiatric hospital. The years you have spent in the cult of your criminal Indian guru have clearly perverted your mind.

You must get professional help and desist with your lies immediately. I will not hesitate to take legal action against you if you choose to persist with your unfounded defamations.

Regards, A.

My hands shake, and my eyes and nose leak as I sob uncontrollably. I can't stand to touch the letter he's written with his filthy hands, and I can't bear for it to be in the house with me, but I may need it as evidence at some future time. Wearing the yellow rubber gloves I use to clean the toilet, I rush into the small backyard, where I dig a hole with a gardening trowel. I wrap the letter in a plastic bag, secure it with tape, place it in the hole and cover it with dirt, determined that no one else will find the letter. I stomp the earth flat with my feet and hope the letter won't poison me from the backyard. Back inside, I pace the floor of the living room and sob with humiliation.

Uncle is right. I am crazy, unstable and a bad person. He will always have all the power, while I'll have none. I want to slice my arms with a knife, but I'm too gutless.

At four in the afternoon, I climb into bed, still with my clothes on. My green sheets are patterned with fluffy white clouds. As I lie on white clouds, I'm in hell. The phone rings and I don't answer. I get up and take four Mersyndol to ease my anguish, crunching them between my teeth so they'll work faster, and I wash the large round pills down with water. Their bitterness matches that of Uncle's letter.

As I get back into bed, I consider that death would be a blessing. If I take all the pills in the house, I might end my suffering, but I could survive and wake up brain damaged. I could jump off the balcony onto the concrete below, but I might survive with permanent injuries instead. I could cut my wrists, but someone will have to clean up all the blood, which would be too traumatic for them. The pills start to work and I feel calmer. I lie on my side in the foetal position and rock my body back and forth to soothe the pain, dozing on and off throughout the long night. My plans of empowerment have come to nought. Robbie was right, the letter was a terrible idea.

As in the game of snakes and ladders, I've tumbled headfirst down a long snake, right back to the bottom. It will take months for me to claw my way, inch by inch, back up the ladder.

The next day, Robbie offers me an emergency appointment. My body shakes as I sit in her room and cry.

'I should have listened to you,' I sob. 'Why didn't I listen to you?'

'I understand your desire for an apology. Don't blame yourself. Most paedophiles don't admit their crimes and are incapable of remorse.'

She hands me a book that will become a constant companion, *Trauma and Recovery* by the psychiatrist Judith Herman.

'I'd like you to read this book so you can better understand perpetrators of abuse. You've suffered a setback, but you *will* find the healing you deserve,' she says gently.

Robbie's book will have a profound impact on me, validating my despair and rage and allowing me to begin to treat myself with compassion and kindness.

CHAPTER SIX

1991

I walk up the stairs for my weekly session with Robbie. With her encouragement, I've been studying social work at Sydney university and am in the second year of my degree. I love learning about social justice and human rights and I've been devouring every library book about feminism I can lay my hands on. Yet I continue to be plagued with fear that I'm too stupid to succeed. Everyone at university is smarter than me. But slowly, I begin to see the world through a new and different lens. The world is larger than my individual trauma and I am developing new friendships. My outlook is expanding. I still feel pain about the past, but I regularly have glimpses of freedom and purpose. This is how I painstakingly build a new and better future.

As I sit with Robbie, I decide to talk with her about my quest to find a mum who loved me.

'Robbie, throughout childhood, I longed to be adopted by a mum who was kind and affectionate, unlike mine, who was depressed, angry or lying down in her room. I was jealous of my friends who had normal mums,' I say sadly.

I go back in time to 1967 when I'm six years old and in my first year of primary school. It's Monday, my favourite day of the week, because school provides safety for the next five days. My brothers and I walk to school to find reprieve from the unhappiness that coats the well-polished furniture and pristine white walls of our home.

My teacher, Fräulein Beckmann, is always predictable and kind.

She's soft and feminine, and wears swishy pastel skirts and mohair cardigans, flesh-coloured stockings and shoes with a heel. Her shiny strawberry-blonde hair is styled into a French bun. I adore everything about her and daydream about living with her.

She gently places her hand on the back of my neck as she walks past me. I wish it were just her and me in the classroom; I don't want to share her with twenty other students. Daydreaming, I imagine her protecting me from Grandpa and Uncle and from our unhappy mother. At school, I pretend extra hard to be cheerful, giggling and joking so everyone will think I'm a happy girl, even though I constantly worry about the dangers that lurk at home.

'Let's open our exercise books and write a story about our weekend,' Fräulein Beckmann says.

'On the weekend, Mum baked a chocolate cake and we went on a picnic in the mountains,' I write.

This is not actually true. Mum stayed in bed for much of the weekend.

'I'm so depressed I can't do anything. You need to make your own dinner,' she told us.

My brother Adrian cooked spaghetti with tomato sauce, sprinkled with a whole packet of parmesan cheese. Dad must have been away on business.

§

After lunch, our class takes a walk along the village creek, where we pick flowers we'll press inside one of the big books that sit on the classroom shelf. In pairs, we hold hands so no one falls into the creek. Fräulein Beckman keeps us safe. She walks just ahead of me, and I watch her straight back longingly. When we return to the classroom, we place our flowers inside the pages of her big book to press them.

She reads us 'Cinderella' from *Grimm's Fairy Tales* and creates different voices for all the characters in the story. I hate Cinderella's mean sisters and stepmum.

Perhaps I could sleep in the classroom until school starts again tomorrow. I'm never scared at school, where there is no danger, no angry voices, no frightening men and no mothers who threaten to kill themselves.

As I sit at my desk with the yellow sunshine streaming through the large windows, I wonder what it would be like to be adopted by Fräulein Beckmann. I picture her cosy house and the bedroom she's furnished just for me, with a bright-orange doona cover and matching pillows, not the depressing brown and beige of my own doona at home. She'll adopt me because I'm her favourite girl and she wants us to be together all the time. I wish I could tell Fräulein Beckman that I'm scared every day, but I remain mute. Since I'm too shy to ask her to adopt me, I try to communicate silently with my eyes, but I don't think she understands my wordless plea.

When I have a new teacher the following year, I hardly ever see Fräulein Beckmann anymore, and I miss her terribly.

§

Three years later in 1970, my best friend Lucie and I walk home from school beneath the bare autumn trees that have lost their golden, brown and orange leaves. We're nine years old. The afternoon light is muted by a cover of grey clouds, and the lights inside the homes are already lit.

Lucie's garden backs onto ours. Her home is a predictable haven away from our unhappy home. We walk through the front door and throw our backpacks on the floor in the hallway.

'You must be hungry,' Lucie's mum says, smiling.

She hugs us both. My body tingles as I melt into her warm bosom. If only I could stay in her embrace forever.

In the kitchen, we devour fizzy lemonade, chocolate biscuits, thick hunks of fresh *Zopf*, a plaited Swiss bread, topped with a generous layer of butter and honey, followed by hot chocolate. I stir five heaped spoons of chocolate powder into my cup, and the milk turns a delicious dark brown.

Lucie's house is messy, with signs of disorder in every room. Her mum isn't a perfect *Hausfrau*, which is why she's so special to me. We make our way upstairs to Lucie's wood-panelled attic room with its sloping ceiling. Her bed is unmade, and I marvel at this act of rebellion. Mum makes our beds every day with tight hospital corners.

'Let's put on some make-up,' Lucie suggests.

We smear each other's lips, cheeks and eyelids with an old box of her mum's make-up. We giggle until our bladders nearly burst. Make-up is magical because Mum doesn't ever wear any. She is a plain woman.

'Let's pretend we are ladies going to a fancy party,' Lucie giggles.

We run downstairs to raid her mum's cupboard. We try on satin dresses and wobble on high heels. We suck on a pencil and blow smoke rings. We're not scared of getting in trouble.

Suddenly, I hear Mum ring the cowbell from across the garden, signalling it's time for me to go home for dinner. A sense of dread quickly grows inside my belly and blooms like a dark ink stain. I want to tell Lucie's mum about the fear I live with every day. I want to ask her to let me live with her and Lucie. But the words stay stuck in my throat because I know Mum's rules: Don't talk, don't tell!

'Bye, Frau Koechlin, thank you for having me.' I smile.

'You're welcome any time, darling.' Lucie's mum embraces me and kisses my cheeks.

As I begin my slow walk home and climb over the garden fence, there is a stone of dread inside my body, making my legs heavy and tired. I wonder what sort of mood Mum is in. Perhaps she'll soon lie down in her darkened bedroom, after taking some sedative pills. She might be silent and withdrawn or perhaps scream at the top of her voice. My steps become slower.

I arrive at the back door, take off my shoes and tippy toe into the immaculate white living room. There's not a speck of dust; nothing is out of order. The black glass table sparkles; the white rug and couch are pristine. I hate the cold grey abstract painting on the wall. Mum is in the kitchen. Reading the tenor of the banging noises she makes, I quickly decide she's angry.

'Hi, Mum, how was your day?' I fawn.

'Set the table, Martina,' she replies.

When Mum, my brothers and I sit down to our dinner in silence, I feel disgusted at the noises my brother David makes as he eats across from me.

§

In 1972, I sit alone on the train from Basel to Schaffhausen, a small town near the centre of Switzerland. Through the train window, I watch as green farms and black-and-white milking cows rush by. Today, for the first time, I've been given permission to take the train on my own. Scared and excited, my heart beats rapidly inside my chest.

Our former nanny, Angelika, lives in Schaffhausen. She took care of and lived with us, when Mum had a bout of severe depression. Angelika is a kindergarten teacher, and I adore every little thing about her. She loves and cuddles me and always makes me laugh.

As the train rushes towards her cosy apartment, my body thrills with joy as I contemplate spending a whole week with her.

Her round face and red cheeks welcome me as I step onto the station platform. She hugs me tightly with her soft body, and we walk home to her tiny apartment, where we sleep at right angles on orange couches that turn into beds at night. In the dark, I feel deep respite inside my stomach and a sense of safety and warmth spreads throughout my body. Angelika is mine for a whole week.

The next day, we meet her friend Regula at the local pool. Lying on the grass between them, I listen as children squeal and splash in the large blue pool. Hanging on Angelika and Regula's every word, I listen to them discuss clothes and diets and make plans for their upcoming summer holiday in Italy. Future husbands are always a favourite topic of conversation.

'Has Bruno called you?' Regula asks.

'Yes, we're going to dinner and a concert next week. I can't believe he likes me.' Angelika giggles.

Jealous, I hate Bruno already, even though I haven't met him. For the thousandth time, I pray for Angelika to adopt me, hoping her future will always include me. She grew up motherless in an orphanage and her mission to find a husband and have five children is easy to understand.

That night, when we lie in our beds, I find the courage to ask her.

'I really want to come and live with you. I'll help you with your babies and the cooking and cleaning. I'll be so good you won't even know I'm there,' I tell her.

'*Liebling*, you already have a family. When I have my babies, you'll be able to visit all the time and you'll be a great help to me,' she replies kindly.

I lie in the dark as silent tears of rejection slide onto the pillow.

The next day, when Angelika is in the basement doing laundry, Bruno rings. I pick up the phone.

'She's not here. I don't know when she'll be home,' I lie.

'Please tell her I called.' Bruno's voice is friendly.

I decide I do hate him. When Angelika returns, I don't tell her about Bruno's phone call. For now, she's all mine.

§

By the time I'm twelve, I stay away as often as possible and spend weekend nights at Lucie's house. On a rainy Saturday, we knit jumpers while we play our favourite music: Cat Stevens, Joni Mitchell, Bob Dylan and Neil Young.

Using a dictionary, we translate the lyrics from English into German. The words evoke a sweet ache within – the promise of belonging and love. My favourite song is 'Sad Lisa' by Cat Stevens. It's as if he intimately knows my pain and speaks directly to me.

'I'm going to marry Cat Stevens when I'm eighteen,' I shout. 'I love his big brown eyes and curly hair.'

'And I'll marry Bob Dylan!' Lucie giggles.

'I've read everything about Cat Stevens. He has a Greek father and Swedish mother and lives in London. I can't wait till we're together,' I say.

'I'll probably live in America with Bob,' Lucie says.

We talk about the long-distance phone calls Lucie and I will have every day and about our lives with our famous husbands with whom we'll tour the world. We don't care about the age difference.

Later, as I lie beside Lucie in her bed, I realise she's drifted off to sleep. The light from the streetlamp shines through the windows. I'm wide awake as I think about my problem. I don't want to go home, and I can't wait six years to marry Cat. Once again, I daydream about Lucie's mum adopting me and I work out that Lucie's room is big enough for both of us. My behaviour will be perfect so that Frau Koechlin will always be pleased to live with me.

Yet I don't have the courage to tell Lucie's mum about my family secrets. I'm too ashamed to admit what life at home is like. The slamming doors, the frightening silences, being hit on our bare bottom with the cane carpet beater, the threats of suicide. Unable to sleep, I toss and turn while Lucie dreams beside me.

All my plans for rescue over the past seven years have come to naught, and I remain trapped.

§

'I wish I'd had a happy mum who was affectionate,' I cry in Robbie's counselling room.

'As a child, you needed your mother to provide consistent love. With your needs unmet, you felt alone in an unpredictable and toxic family system. You needed your mother and father's protection, but instead you were exposed to abuse by paedophiles, and your parents looked the other way. Your mother was a source of overwhelming distress, and your father was absent. You were harmed repeatedly in childhood, including through emotional, physical and sexual abuse. The constant stress you endured explains your search for a mum who might adopt and keep you safe. Your childish fantasies lessened your pain.' Robbie's eyes are full of compassion.

By now, I've shed so many tears, they might cover the floor of her room.

'I'm lucky I had safe women in my childhood – my primary school teacher, Fräulein Beckmann, Lucie's mum, Frau Koechlin, and Angelika,' I sigh. 'And I have you now.'

'In time, you'll learn to become your own tender mother. You can nurture your inner child with the kindness you always longed for. Let's try it now. Picture putting little Martina on your lap and hugging her with love,' Robbie suggests.

In my imagination, I kiss little Martina's face and wipe away her tears. I tell her I will always cherish and keep her safe. I gently hold her hands and stroke them.

On my way home, I feel a new sense of peace and lightness. There were people who loved me when I was a child and I wasn't completely alone.

CHAPTER SEVEN

1992

Heavy rains buffet the car as I drive to my therapy session on a Monday morning. The windscreen wipers are on their fastest setting and the windscreen is fogged up. The traffic has slowed to a crawl with the storm and I'm worried I'll be late for my appointment. While waiting at a red light, I decide to tell Robbie about becoming a thief when I was ten years old. I feel embarrassed, but I know by now that honesty in therapy is essential if I want to heal. Out of breath, I arrive at Robbie's office and take off my raincoat. The room is cosy, and I instantly feel safe in her calm presence.

'I need to tell you something embarrassing.' I look at the floor, avoiding eye contact.

'Go ahead, Martina, you know this is a judgement-free zone.' Robbie smiles.

In the therapy room, I go back in time to my childhood kitchen. I'm stuffing a hunk of Mum's home-baked bread into my mouth, slathered with an extra thick layer of butter and honey.

'How many times do I have to tell you to dry the dishes?' Mum yells.

When I grab the tea towel to dry the dishes that are stacked in the dish rack, a thrilling idea suddenly enters my mind. I know where Mum keeps her purse, so today I'm going to steal money from her because she's such a mean and horrible mum. With the money, I'll buy some chocolate at the corner shop.

Mum keeps her leather purse in the left-hand drawer of the red Formica kitchen bench where she also keeps pens, rubber bands, sticky tape and her shopping list. When Mum goes to the bathroom, I quietly slide open the kitchen drawer, take out her purse and quickly check its contents. I'm too scared to steal bank notes, but there are plenty of coins waiting for me. I grab a five-franc and a two-franc coin, a small fortune, and put them in the pocket of my gym shorts. I return the wallet and silently slide the drawer shut. My heart pounds with excitement, and when Mum comes back, I do my best to look innocent as I keep drying the dishes. The money in my pocket gives me a thrilling sense of happiness.

On my way to school the next day, I stop at the corner shop and buy my favourite creamy hazelnut chocolate and a small bottle of Coca-Cola – a new fizzy drink from America that is forbidden at home. I also buy the yellow exercise book covered in rainbows, in which I plan to write my secrets. I'll hide it beneath the winter jumpers in the back of my wardrobe. I'm exhilarated by my secret purchases.

As soon as I leave the little shop, I tear open the block of chocolate and stuff it into my mouth. Savouring the sweet chocolate, I allow it to melt in my mouth. Chomping on the hazelnuts, I crunch them between my teeth. I desperately need this sweetness, since there's none to be found at home. Opening the glass bottle of Coca-Cola, I relish its fizzy tang. Transported to a place of pure pleasure, some of the cola dribbles onto my red t-shirt, leaving a dark stain.

I've just discovered a new trifecta of happiness: freedom from pain, secret rebellion and sweet revenge. Stealing Mum's money becomes a satisfying act of dissent. From this day on, I will continue to take money from Mum's purse – and soon also from Dad's trouser pockets, which hang on the hook on the back of my parents' dressing room door at night.

'Do you think I'm a bad person, stealing money from Mum and Dad?' I ask Robbie.

'Many children take money from their parents – it's a way of searching for the love they're missing, and at the same time, a silent form of punishment for the love they've been denied,' Robbie explains. She doesn't judge me.

'Let's explore how you can now offer your inner child the love she was once denied. This will be far more healing than taking money from your parents. Your inner child longs for your kindness. You had many harmful experiences in childhood, Martina. You cried out for help, but no one was listening. No one kept you safe or attended to your pain. Instead, everyone looked the other way. Now you have the chance to heal your wounded child by creating a safe inner and outer environment. By listening to and honouring your inner child, you can provide her the safety and security you needed back then. If you do this consistently, the positive traits of your inner child will have room to shine,' Robbie explains.

Her suggestion sounds strange to me, but I'm desperate enough to give it a try.

'I want to teach you how to find your very own safe place, where you can find shelter in your imagination, when things become overwhelming in- and outside the therapy room. Close your eyes and allow an image of your special safe place to come to you,' Robbie instructs me.

I settle into the armchair, watching the rain fall and the liquid amber tree swaying outside the window, as the sound of the storm fills the room. I close my eyes and search for a place where I felt happy and safe in the past. An image comes to me.

'Robbie, my safe place is called "Plaine Madeleine" – a field of green. A creek runs through it. It's in the mountains, where I used to spend my childhood holidays.' I smile knowing Grandpa and Uncle never visited my special place.

I tell Robbie that my safe place is fringed by a forest of fragrant larch- and pine trees. Snow-capped mountains surround us, and I smell the earthy cinnamon of tiny mountain flowers.

'Grandpa and Uncle can't hurt me there,' I tell Robbie as my stomach relaxes and my breath slows and deepens.

'It sounds very beautiful. Can you tell me more? Let yourself become fully immersed in this place and picture yourself as the precious little girl you were. How old are you in your safe place?'

'I'm six years old and I'm lying on a picnic blanket beside a small creek.' The tension in my body melts away, and I feel a profound sense of calm.

I listen to the sound of the water that journeys down all the way from the mountain glaciers and cup my hands to drink the icy cold blue liquid. The sun warms my body and a gentle breeze ruffles the long grass. I pick my favourite flower, a small purple bloom that has the delicious fragrance of rich dark chocolate.

In the counselling room, the scent of chocolate fills the air, causing my breathing and body to relax even further.

I watch a pair of mountain goats with their curled horns, and there are marmot babies playing and tumbling together. On her hind legs, their mum makes sure they are safe.

'It's so peaceful. I hope Grandpa and Uncle will never find me here,' I say.

'What do you need to feel even safer?' Robbie asks me.

'I need Basil.' Basil is my first dog, who has recently come into my life, an energetic kelpie with intelligent amber eyes, black silky fur and large pointy ears.

'Picture Basil beside you, Martina. Feel his safe presence,' Robbie instructs me.

'Basil is leaning against me, panting. He's protecting me from danger.'

Suddenly, my paedophiles appear in my safe place and in the counselling room and I grip the arms of the chair tightly.

'Robbie, they've come to hurt me. Grandpa's face is angry and I'm scared he'll hit me with his walking stick. Uncle is also here. They want to punish me for talking about them. Why have they come?' I cry.

'What do you need to do to keep your inner child safe from harm?' Robbie asks.

'I need Basil to protect me. He's just developed magic powers. He's turning into a ferocious beast, twice the size of a lion. He growls and barks; his fangs are huge and scary.' I smile.

'I'll protect you, Martina,' he barks. 'Don't be scared anymore. They won't hurt you ever again.'

'Robbie, Basil is hunting them down. He catches Grandpa and Uncle, who are hiding behind some trees. Basil is snarling; he wants their blood. They run from him and cry out for help.' I giggle.

But there is no one to help them. Now they know what it was like for me when I was a small child. Basil catches Grandpa first because he's old and slow on his walking stick. Grandpa, that fat bald man, is crying out in agony as Basil bites down hard on his calves and then drags him along the ground. Basil stands above him, while Grandpa begs for mercy. Basil rips Grandpa's shirt and bites his flabby white stomach, causing him to cry out in agony. Blood oozes from Grandpa's stomach. His internal organs are spilling out.

'Grandpa is helpless against Basil's fangs.' I giggle.

'I'm sorry, please forgive me!' Grandpa begs.

But Basil shows no mercy. While Grandpa lies dying, Basil hunts down Uncle, the worst of my perpetrators. Basil pounces on him and drags Uncle along the ground. He pulls out large chunks of his thick black hair, leaving bleeding bald patches. He rips Uncle's clothes and rolls him over onto his stomach. He grabs him by the neck and violently shakes it back and forth.

'He's breaking Uncle's neck; bright red blood is gushing everywhere.' I laugh.

Sweet delight at this revenge fills me.

'I'm sorry, so sorry!' Uncle begs for mercy.

'Robbie, they're both terrified. They're even apologising,' I giggle.

Joy runs up and down my body in delicious waves.

'Do you think I'm a bad person for having these fantasies? Is it wrong to imagine revenge?' I ask Robbie.

'No, it's not wrong. As human beings, we have permission to entertain any thought we want. We can't act on every thought, but our imagination allows us true freedom. You're a strong young woman with the courage to defend yourself against the crimes that were committed against you. Your imagination is entirely your own. You have every right to be angry and to envision taking revenge. In this way, you're discovering your worth and dignity, and empowering yourself to stand up to the relatives who harmed you. This is how you're learning to heal your inner child. I'm very proud of you.' Robbie's smile is warm and reassuring.

I'm relieved she's not judging me. Once Basil has punished the perpetrators and rendered them powerless, he returns to his normal size and snuggles into my body; his soft warm black fur brings deep comfort. The perpetrators have disappeared, and we lie once again together on the soft green grass. Basil's heartbeat soothes the very core of my being.

I put my arms around him and tell him, 'You're a good boy, Basil!'

As I drive home after the session, I smile with pleasure. I'm a strong woman, able to protect myself from the memories of those who harmed me. Now that I feel safe, I know they'll never be able to hurt me again, and my future holds the promise of hope and healing.

CHAPTER EIGHT

1992

A few weeks later, I'm once again sitting with Robbie in her counselling room. She has become the most significant person in my life, supporting me on my path of healing. Her kindness and wisdom guide me towards safety. My former guru had promised a cure that never came to pass and my eight long years of devotion only led to deeper wounds. Heavy winter winds rattle the windowpanes of the counselling room, making it difficult for us to hear each other. I'm ashamed to tell Robbie about being harmed by two more people.

'I need to tell you about the two boys who also sexually abused me. Do you think I had a sign on my forehead saying, "Abuse me?" Was I asking for it?' I ask.

'No, Martina, you were vulnerable to further abuse because you weren't protected by your caregivers,' Robbie replies gently.

'I'm ten years old, and Paul is in the class above me,' I say.

I explain to her that Paul has recently moved into the new architect-designed concrete and glass mansion in our cul-de-sac. His house has an indoor swimming pool and a real electric lift, as well as a red Ferrari in the garage.

'Do you want to come over after school?' Paul asks. 'We have lots of Coca-Cola.'

In awe of his fancy new home and excited about the Coca-Cola, we go to his place after school.

In our undies, we swim in the heated indoor pool and take trips up and down in the three-storey lift. I've never been in a lift before. I don't meet his parents or older brothers. It's as if he lives there alone and unsupervised, already a grown-up.

After about a couple of hours, I hear Mum ring the cowbell, calling me home for dinner.

'I have to go home right away,' I tell Paul urgently. I'll be in trouble if I'm late for dinner.

As I approach the front door, he places his large body in front of it, blocking me from leaving. His eyes have become menacing. I realise he is much bigger and stronger than me, and he can smell my fear.

'You can't leave until you've done as I tell you to do,' he hisses.

I must lick his bum hole and his penis, and he will do the same to me.

'If you don't do it, I'll take you hostage and you'll never see your family again,' he threatens.

I freeze. I have no choice because I'll be in trouble if I don't get home in the next five minutes, so I squeeze my eyes shut and obey him, even though the act fills me with unbearable shame. His smell is disgusting, and I have an overpowering urge to vomit. As soon as he's finished with me, I pull my pants up and run out of that terrible house.

When I get home, I scrub my mouth and hands and sit at the dinner table, my face a mask hiding my deep shame. This experience marks yet another secret I must never reveal.

'Robbie, I wonder how a boy thinks of such a degrading game. Is it my fault?' I ask her, crying.

'You mustn't blame yourself, Martina. You were a child, trained to obey those who harmed you. You didn't stand a chance against Paul. Have you heard of the term victim-blaming? It's the prevalent societal belief that victims are "asking for it", that they want to be harmed and that the abuse is therefore their own fault. It's a convenient belief that protects perpetrators and allows them to get away with their crimes.' Robbie gazes at me with kindness, her voice firm.

My stomach relaxes, my heart slows and gratitude fills my body as I take in Robbie's words. It's not my fault that I was abused and, with her help, I'm learning to put the blame where it belongs.

'Next time I'll tell you about the other boy who hurt me,' I say.

'Yes, please tell me. There is nothing we can't talk about,' she reminds me.

§

The following week, I take a seat in the armchair across from Robbie. My right leg pumps rapidly up and down and shame overwhelms me once again. Avoiding eye contact, I look down at the richly patterned rug beneath me.

When I'm fourteen, our family moves to Australia because Dad gets an exciting job offer. When we arrive there, I'm swallowed by a constant sense of foreignness, and the ache of homesickness runs deep. I miss my friends – especially Lucie – as well as my native language and the comforting foods of home. I meet Jorge, a seventeen-year-old boy who goes to school down the road. He's three years older; he's in Year Twelve while I'm in Year Eight. He has recently moved to Australia from Argentina with his parents and three little sisters. He has an exotic accent, a black afro, olive skin, a cool leather jacket and a Yamaha 125 motorbike. He asks me to go see *One Flew Over the Cuckoo's Nest* with him at Hoyts cinema in Sydney's George Street. We share popcorn and sip Coke at the movies, trading stories about everything we miss from home and how bland and dull Australia feels in comparison.

'I'm not looking for a girlfriend,' he tells me. 'Let's just be friends.'

I tell him that's fine with me. As we watch Jack Nicholson challenge the strict rules of the psychiatric hospital he is locked up in, Jorge starts touching my breasts. He hugs me too hard and won't release me. There's no tenderness – just groping hands, careless and suffocating. No one has taught me yet about power and consent. In fact, I have by now been fundamentally groomed to be an obedient girl. At fourteen, my breasts are already large, but psychologically I'm still a child, while he is a young man with copious amounts of testosterone. I can't make sense of what's happening in the darkness of the cinema. He is meant to be a friend to me, yet he's crossing boundaries I don't know how to name.

The next day, Jorge waits for me after school and, all too quickly, I start to dread seeing him because he only wants one thing. I wish I knew what to say. I'd stop seeing him – but I just can't find the words. This is how I remain trapped with Jorge for nearly a year of relentless sexual harassment. I detest the sexual attacks I endure in parks, in our garage and at his house. When I'm away from Jorge, I tell myself how lucky I am that he is my friend. But when I'm with him, his body overwhelms mine, just like what happened when I was a much smaller child.

On a balmy summer evening, Jorge picks me up after dinner and we ride to a nearby park. I sit on the back of his motorbike and put my arms around his waist. I'm feeling glamorous as the wind tumbles my hair which I'm growing into a long bob with a fringe, like Joni Mitchell. Jorge parks the motorbike and finds a secluded spot in the park beneath a Morton Bay fig. We lie in its shade and he forces his tongue into my mouth. My body quickly goes into shutdown, and I can't breathe. His arms pin me down, and he transforms into a monster – just like Grandpa and Uncle.

He sucks on my neck and breasts – a vampire leaving angry dark-red marks that turn purple and, over time, blue and yellow.

He doesn't notice – or doesn't care – that my body is pleading for him to stop. No longer present, I dissociate and, light as a balloon, fly to the top of the Morton Bay fig, from where I look down at a scene that makes me gag. I wish I had the courage to get up and walk away from Jorge. Later, he drives me home. He's in a tender mood, while I'm dirty and ashamed, an injured fourteen-year-old without a voice.

That night I lie in bed, unable to sleep. Thinking through my options, I wonder how I might rescue myself from the trap I've found myself in. I long to be free of Jorge, but the idea of telling him out loud seems impossible. Perhaps I could ask Mum to help me. I could tell her about the things he's been doing to me. But these acts are unspeakable, and she'll probably blame and punish me. Finally, I have the idea that I could write him a letter. Quickly choosing this option, I turn on the bedside light and pull out a page of my notebook.

Dear Jorge, I don't think we should spend time together anymore. I am sorry, Martina.

Relief floods my body and the rock of fear inside my stomach softens. I sneak into Dad's study and take a stamp and envelope from his desk drawer, on which I write Jorge's name and address. Eventually I go to sleep, certain my nightmare is about to end. I'll post the letter on my way to school; after that, I'll finally be free of Jorge's attacks.

Two days later while I'm doing my maths homework after school, the doorbell rings. When I open the front door, Jorge is standing there holding my letter. His body is shaking with sobs. This isn't what's supposed to happen. We go into the back garden and he hugs me so hard I can't breathe.

'I love you and I can't live without you. I'm going to kill myself if you leave me,' he sobs.

I'm confused. He said we were just friends but now he's saying he loves me. Without a fight, I surrender. If he's so distraught, I don't have the right to say no to him. His needs trump mine. I can't admit how much I dread the sex – it feels like it's the only part of me he values, and without it, he might kill himself. This is how I remain entrapped. It takes several more months before I can finally break free from Jorge – and this only happens when I meet my first real boyfriend, our next-door neighbour Toby, who tells Jorge to leave me alone.

'Robbie, what's wrong with me?' I whisper. 'I wish I'd been stronger.'

'Whose fault was Jorge's abuse? Who had more power?' Robbie asks. Her face is full of care, but her voice is firm once again.

'He was three years older; that's a big age difference. If he'd cared enough to notice, he would have known I hated the things he made me do.' I can't stop weeping.

'Children who experience sexual abuse are five times more likely to be assaulted again,' Robbie explains. 'The age at which a child's abuse first occurs influences the risk of future victimisation. Those abused before the age of twelve are especially vulnerable. Offenders often sense and exploit this vulnerability, making survivors more frequent targets.'

'Yes,' I say, blowing my nose. 'That is exactly what happened to me in childhood. I was abused by my relatives and I didn't stand a chance against Paul and Jorge. Also, I'd only just moved to Australia and was homesick and lost.'

Robbie has a way of saying exactly what I need to hear, allowing me to experience a gradually increasing kindness and forgiveness towards myself. Slowly, I'm beginning to see things in a new and different light. The abuse is not my shame, but that of my perpe-trators. I'm also beginning to tap into the potent force of anger toward my paedophiles, and with it comes a renewed sense of strength and empowerment.

Each time I leave a session with Robbie, I'm energised and hopeful that I'm building a new life of dignity and worth. Now in my third year of university, I finally believe I'm smart enough to succeed. I'm setting boundaries, as well as forming meaningful friendships with women. I have left behind the years of abuse, as well as the blind faith I had in a fraudulent guru.

CHAPTER NINE

1992

On my way to my Monday morning session with Robbie, my stomach is bloated and sore after yesterday's food binge, and I've put on my loosest dress to conceal my distended belly. I decide I must confess the secret about my body shame that is as insistent as the noise of cicadas on a hot summer's day, a constant clamour defeating me with its cruel voice, telling me I'm fat and disgusting.

'Robbie, I hate my body.' I cry with exhaustion, my stomach painfully swollen.

I'm too embarrassed to tell her I weigh myself several times a day, and when I get out of bed, I walk backwards so my boyfriend won't see my big fat bum.

'Almost every minute of the day, I obsess about how much I weigh, what I've eaten, what I shouldn't have eaten and whether I've been *good* or *bad*,' I cry.

'Many sexual abuse survivors develop eating disorders. Your body is where the abuse took place, so you mistrust it and are at war with it,' Robbie explains.

'I drink coffee and smoke cigarettes all day. I allow myself only one meal in the evening. Otherwise, I'll get too fat.' I'm relieved to admit the truth to her.

'I'm going to help you learn to eat three meals a day. Your body and brain need regular meals, or you'll stay compliant and disempowered,' Robbie says, looking worried.

'But I also binge on chocolate, pastries, ice cream, bread, pizza and chips. I binged all day yesterday. After each binge, I'm disgusted with myself,' I sob.

Robbie hands me her box of tissues.

'When we chronically undereat, the pendulum always swings back, causing us to binge eat. The bingeing is a direct result of starvation. When you start to feed your body regularly, the bingeing will settle. Also, your preoccupation with your body provides a distraction from the things that lie beneath body shame. For example, your anguish about your sexual abuse.' Robbie smiles reassuringly.

She consistently helps me uncover the truth that lies hidden beneath my conscious awareness.

'Ninety per cent of my thoughts revolve around food and my weight,' I tell Robbie.

'The pursuit of thinness causes women endless highs and lows, heartache and despair. In this way, body shame has become your intimate companion. Perhaps you're blaming your body instead of your abusers.' Robbie's grey eyes are patient.

I go back in time to being twelve and standing at the fridge, shovelling honey yoghurt into my mouth and savouring its creamy sweetness. Mum watches me from her wicker chair, her glasses perched low on her nose and her mouth frowning. She has curlers in her hair, covered with a yellow hairnet, and she's still in her light blue dressing gown.

'Your bum is too fat. Come with me, I'll weigh you,' she instructs.

I've never thought about my bum before. Walking with her into the bathroom, I step on the scales.

'Just as I thought, you are getting fat. Your BMI is twenty-four,' Mum says as she consults her book on how to achieve thinness.

I don't know what a BMI is. Mum takes out her tape measure from the bathroom drawer and measures my chest, waist and hips, and shakes her head disapprovingly, the corners of her mouth turned down.

'Your hips are too big. I'm putting you on a diet. One thousand calories a day will get you down to a BMI of twenty,' she tells me, because she is an expert on weight loss. After she's weighed and measured me, Mum steps on the scales and shares her defeat with me.

'I've gained half a kilo but I've been so good. How did this happen?' Mum moans.

She tells me she hates her legs, that they're thick like hundred-year-old oak trees, and that her cellulite is disgusting.

When she sits down to breakfast, she allows herself only one soft-boiled egg. She taps the top of the egg with a spoon and eats it slowly, adding salt and pepper to each bite.

'I've just eaten sixty-three calories so that's all I'll have until dinner.' She stirs fake sweetener into her black coffee and takes a small sip.

§

Over the next couple of years, Mum and I go on the grapefruit diet, the Israeli diet, Weight Watcher's, the egg diet, the Doctor Atkins diet and juice fasting. I quickly become Mum's willing apprentice in the quest to free ourselves of our shameful curves. The pursuit of shrinking ourselves, to have control over our thighs, stomach and hips becomes the glue that unites us. I desperately want to shrink my large breasts that remain the constant focus of the male gaze. By the time I'm thirteen, I know by heart the calorie value of every food.

But it's boring to stick to a diet day after day. I miss the forbidden foods that provide such reliable comfort. One day, I research the number of calories in a block of chocolate. It has one thousand calories – exactly what I'm allowed to eat in a day. I yearn for the sweetness of chocolate, so I steal some money from Mum's wallet, buy a block of milk chocolate and nibble on it throughout the day.

'I'm sick, Mum. I won't eat any dinner,' I tell her. In my room, I lie on the bed reading and allow the sweetness of the chocolate to comfort me.

Back in the counselling room, I cry tears of relief, having finally admitted to Robbie the cruel ways I treat my body. I *want* to learn to love my body, but I don't want to get fat if I eat three meals a day, as Robbie is proposing. I pretend to go along with her suggestions, but I secretly vow to only increase my daily intake of food to two small meals a day. It will take me several more years to consistently eat three meals with regular snacks, and to trust that my body will eventually settle into its natural, comfortable state.

CHAPTER TEN

1992

Despite weekly counselling sessions, the sexual abuse continues to affect me. As I sit in Robbie's steadfast presence, I'm furious that decades later – and after three years of therapy – I'm still overwhelmed by the impact of sexual abuse.

'The abuse is the gift that keeps on giving, a gift I never asked for,' I say bitterly. 'My grandfather and uncle have robbed me of a stable life. I just want to feel normal.' I rip at my cuticles that are red and throbbing from the harm I've inflicted on them over the past days.

'Yes, your relatives *have* robbed you. No one has been more committed to healing, and yet here you are, still suffering. Your recovery from abuse will take longer than you imagined, but I promise that you will feel better in time,' Robbie reassures me.

She is wearing a blue linen dress, which matches her eyes, and her beautifully lined face reveals the story of her life, a story I'll never know. Confident she will guide me with care and expertise throughout our session, I feel held in her presence.

I go back once more to my grandparents' house.

'Mum is in the dining room, and Grandpa is shouting at her,' I say, sobbing.

He stands threateningly over Mum, massive in a black suit and tie, while I watch them from the hallway and hold my breath. I suddenly see Mum's beige pants as they become stained. Mum has wet her pants. A dark patch spreads down her thighs. She looks terrified. Crying, she suddenly runs out of the house, gets in her car and drives away without me.

'Mum was also scared of Grandpa. I'm sorry for her, but I can't believe she left me behind.' I wipe at my tears with the back of my hand.

'Return to that scene, Martina, and see what else you notice.' Robbie's voice is soft and comforting.

I go back to a time later that day. I'm on the first floor in the bathroom. Grandma has run me a bath. Surrounded by bubbles, I play with yellow rubber ducks. The bubbles smell of lavender, just like Grandma does. I try to play like a normal child, but my ears are finely tuned, scanning for danger.

'I'm in the bath and Uncle's just come into the bathroom.' I hyperventilate and my body shakes.

'Take some slow breaths, Martina. Remember you are safe here in Australia, far away from your abusers,' Robbie instructs.

'But he's here,' I cry. 'He's leaning down and touching me. His fingers are like snakes and his cleft chin is horrible.' I bite the inside of my cheek.

I experience a throbbing pain between my legs.

'I can feel him on me.' I sob, a heartbroken child.

'What can you do to help little Martina?' Robbie asks.

'My adult self has come into the bathroom. I pick little Martina up and hold her in my arms. I kiss the top of her head and wrap a towel around her,' I tell Robbie.

She's such a sweet girl, so small and vulnerable. I put on her pink pyjamas. She puts her head on my shoulder and wraps her little arms and legs around me. I carry her out of that terrible house. My car is out the front and I strap her in her child seat, while Basil sits next to her and gives her kisses. She squeals with delight and soon they cuddle up and fall asleep together. We drive through the dark streets to Basel airport, where we board a plane for Australia.' I smile.

'What do you want to say to little Martina?'

'You never have to go back to that house, sweetheart. I'll always keep you safe,' I tell her, stroking her forehead.

On the plane, I cover her with a soft blanket, and she curls up in my lap and falls asleep. In this way, I'm learning to care tenderly for little Martina and repair the damage that was done to me.

'You've worked hard today, Martina,' Robbie says with a smile, her eyes full of compassion.

Back in the counselling room, I'm lighter than when I walked in. I've survived, and there *is* hope. Therapy is helping me overcome the pain of the past, and I'm proud of my courage today. I drink deeply from the glass of water Robbie hands me.

As I drive home, my mouth throbs where I bit the inside of my cheeks during the worst of today's memories. I stop at a red light and place my left hand on my heart, grateful I'm developing the capacity to take care of my sad inner child. There are many children inside me, each embodying a different stage of childhood. This afternoon, my inner child is a four-year-old, abused in the bathtub by her uncle.

Grateful Robbie is teaching me to care for myself, I'm learning to soothe the wounds that have been inflicted on me. Robbie helps me mother the child that didn't receive comfort. Mum didn't know how to keep me safe. I can't have a different mum, but I can be a good mum to myself.

'I'm proud of you, darling,' I tell the small girl inside as the light turns green and I release the handbrake and put my foot on the accelerator. I love talking to her like this. She trusts me and tells me she feels happy with me. She calls me Mama. I call her my darling and sweetheart and hunny bun, pet names I was never called. In my imagination, I hug her the way I yearned to be cuddled in childhood.

My inner child is many things: adorable, needy, scared, jealous, sweet and angry. I bring care to all her manifestations. I offer her my full acceptance and heartfelt compassion, no matter what she's going through.

PART THREE:
RISING

CHAPTER ONE

1992

'I have a big D on my forehead,' I tell Robbie.

'What's a D?' she asks.

'Damaged goods!' I roll my eyes.

It's the middle of winter and there's a violent storm outside the warm safety of the counselling room. Branches from the liquid amber tree scratch against the windowpanes, and the wind howls. Robbie has lit a candle, and we sip cups of fragrant green tea. She looks at me through her horn-rimmed glasses; her gaze makes me feel cared for. Today is the start of many talks with Robbie about love. About what I do and don't want as a single thirty-year-old looking for love.

'I want to find love. I think I'm ready. But what if no one will ever love me? What if all men are pricks?' My right foot pumps up and down.

'Let's talk about the signs of a healthy relationship,' Robbie suggests.

'How would I know about that?' I laugh sadly.

At home after the counselling session, I look through my books on co-dependence and study the green and red flags of relationships. From this research, I create my own list of the non-negotiable qualities I will seek in a partner:

- Loyalty
- Seeks commitment

- Is a friend to me
- Speaks respectfully about their ex-partners
- Willing to have difficult conversations
- Cares about social justice
- Does what they say they will do
- Willing to say sorry
- Isn't a regular drinker or drug user
- Compassionate
- Doesn't push for sex
- Values women of all ages
- Has a sense of humour
- Is financially stable
- Doesn't want children.

I stick the list on the fridge as a reminder of my commitment to myself. The list will be my north star, ensuring I won't fall for shitty men anymore.

A few days later, I sit across from Jack at a pizza place in Darlinghurst. I gaze at his long dark eyelashes, curly hair and strong shoulders, which remind me of Robert De Niro. I tell myself not to fall for his looks, to remain focused on my list instead.

'My ex is crazy, totally unhinged,' he tells me as he drinks his red wine in generous gulps.

'How long were you together for?' I ask.

'Ten months. Ten months too long,' he says with a grimace.

He refills his glass and swigs more wine, leaving a red stain around his mouth.

'Are you sure you don't want any?' he asks.

'No thanks, I'm on a bit of a health kick.' I smile.

'What about your ex?'

'We were together on and off for five years. He's a nice guy, but a big drinker and stoner,' I tell Jack.

How I miss my ex. I still look for his white Subaru wherever I go. He drove off in it a year ago, and moved in with a prettier, younger and presumably less fucked-up girlfriend.

'Are you looking for a partner, or just some fun?' I ask Jack.

'God, no, I'm not partner material. I'm *puer eternus*, the eternal adolescent.' He laughs as he pours himself another glass of wine.

'Okay, that's good to know.' I smile at him with my mouth but not with my eyes.

We finish our meal. Although he is on a generous salary as a solicitor and I'm barely able to pay the rent, we go halves.

'Do you want to come back to mine?' he asks when we walk outside.

While tempted and starved for love, I remind myself to pay attention to the red flags. *Come on, Martina, what would Robbie say?*

'Thanks, Jack, but I have an early start tomorrow.' I kiss him on the cheek and walk home by myself.

Maybe my friends who've seen the list on the fridge are right when they tell me I'll never find a partner because I'm too picky. But I remind myself to trust my higher self. Jack will only bring me misery, and I'm okay on my own, so I'll stick to my list.

§

In therapy the next morning, Robbie and I analyse my date with Jack.

'He drank a whole bottle of wine and spoke badly about his ex. That's two red flags,' I tell her.

I'm excited that I stuck to my principles. I'm getting stronger, and this is a new sign of self-respect.

'It's great you've got your list to guide you,' Robbie says.

'He's very good looking, and in the past, I would have definitely gone home with him,' I tell Robbie. Aware that sexual attraction is not the best tool for choosing a mate, I feel proud I listened to my higher self.

'I'm proud of you, too, Martina. You're making big changes that will lead to love that is safe and kind,' Robbie says.

§

One day, Michael, a friend of a friend, invites me for dinner. All I know about him is that he's divorced and doesn't drink.

He picks me up in his small red vintage Alfa Romeo and we drive to North Bondi to have dinner at a restaurant called Sean's Panorama.

The waiter shows us to a table overlooking the ocean. The surf is huge, and we watch the waves as they crash onto the shore. The waiter hands us our menus. The theme that night is all about meat – so the whole menu is packed with meat dishes.

'I'm vegetarian. I don't think there's anything I can eat here,' I say, embarrassed.

'I'll go and sort it out.' Michael smiles and gets up from his chair.

As he walks towards the kitchen, I check out his body. He has strong arms and looks fit. I consider green and red flags. I can already see some green flags and no red flags yet, but the night has only just begun. I tell myself not to be too hopeful and to just observe things with detachment.

'I've organised a vegetarian meal with the chef. Is pumpkin risotto okay for you?'

'I love risotto,' I say with a smile, pleased Michael has taken care of the situation.

We order lemon, lime and bitters.

'You don't drink?' I ask Michael.

'No, I don't. I've been sober from drugs and alcohol for a year.' He smiles, his face open.

'That's cool. Tell me more about that.' I'm tempted to bite my nails but I place my hands on the table instead.

'I got clean and sober when my ex-wife and I split up.' He looks thoughtful. 'I was using a lot of drugs back then.' He takes a sip of his drink.

I like his honesty and willingness to reflect on his behaviour.

After dinner, we walk along Bondi Beach. He is handsome, but not too handsome. I'm comfortable and calm with him rather than hyped up and excited. When he drops me back home, he doesn't grope me, but gives me a kiss on my cheek. I like that a lot.

§

A few weeks later, we take Basil for a walk in Centennial Park.

'I don't want to have sex for the first six months, but I totally get it if that doesn't work for you,' I tell him, feeling shy.

I probably won't see him after this walk. He'll get in his car and drive away, thinking I'm a nut.

'I like that idea. There's no rush,' he says calmly.

§

A few weeks later, we are lying on my bed talking. We gaze at each other; his blue-grey eyes tell me he is completely present. We hold hands and kiss slowly, our bodies touching, but we don't have sex. This is an entirely new experience. Finally, I'm gifted the innocent adolescence that was stolen from me by my perpetrators.

'I'd like to get married someday, but I don't want kids and I'll

153

never be a wife who does all the housework,' I say, worried he'll think I'm being too bossy.

'I don't think I want kids either, and I love grocery shopping and doing laundry. I also make a great pumpkin soup.' He smiles and kisses my forehead.

When he drops me off at university that afternoon, I walk across the lawns to my lecture. I suddenly experience a sharp pain in my chest. The sensation is so overwhelming that I lie down on the grass to catch my breath. Certain I'm having a heart attack, I miss my lecture. Sweat pools in my armpits and on my forehead, and my head spins as I suddenly realise I might be in the middle of falling in love with Michael. My hands are clammy, and I hyperventilate. I could get hurt again and I can't stand to feel this vulnerable. Love is terrifying.

§

In the months after we fall in love, the previously hidden parts of me – my fears, my wounds – start to surface, ugly and unruly. I pick fights with Michael as my childhood traumas emerge in terrifying succession. Convinced that Michael will leave me or cheat on me, my behaviour becomes deplorable and I threaten to break up with him over the smallest disagreements.

One day, we're swimming with my five-year-old godchildren, the twins Sarah and Josh, in their pool. Michael is throwing them up in the air, and they scream in delight, while I watch like a hawk. Is he touching their genitals under the water? I dive down and watch his hands on their small bodies, suddenly convinced he's a paedophile like Grandpa and Uncle.

Another day, we argue. He's at my place and is laughing on the phone with his friend Leo, but has been distant and quiet towards me, leaving me feeling insecure and needy. I'm certain he's losing interest in me and that he'll soon break up with me. In that instant, I cover my fear with anger and turn into a woman just like Mum, my fury explosive.

'You're nice to Leo but you treat me like shit!' I yell, convinced he doesn't love me anymore.

He looks at me, confused.

'I know exactly what's going on!' I shout.

I'm certain he wants to leave me, though apart from being a little withdrawn, there's no proof of this.

'What are you talking about?' He shakes his head at me and frowns.

Overcome with rage, I grab the television remote control and hit him on the head with all my strength. Blood drips from the top of his head.

'I can't believe you just did that,' he says, protecting his head with his hands.

He walks out the door, gets in his car and drives away.

Ashamed and terrified, I sit on the floor and shake. I try to phone him but he doesn't pick up. I'm a hypocrite. I want a man who is comfortable with his emotions, but I'm unable to regulate my own. I seek commitment, but I threaten to leave during our slightest disagreement. I need him to have difficult conversations in a calm way, yet I lash out in anger, unable to discuss things reasonably. I want a partner who isn't a regular drinker or drug user, but I secretly continue to numb myself with pills.

I keep calling him until he finally picks up the phone.

'This isn't working for me. I won't accept abuse,' he says, his voice firm.

'I'm so sorry. I don't want to lose you, Michael. I'll be better,' I promise, feeling desperate.

Michael talks to me about safety and respect, while I sit on the floor and cry.

'Okay, I'll give you one last chance.' Michael's tone is firm and I know he means it.

'Please God, help me be better,' I whisper after I put down the phone, tears running down my face. I'm so ashamed.

§

A few days later, I attend a lecture on childhood development. As the lecturer talks about attachment theory, it's as if she's speaking directly to me. According to attachment theory, I developed a potent mix of anxious and avoidant attachment in early childhood, called disorganised attachment. Tears of sorrow and relief smudge the ink on my notepad. Since Mum and Dad were unable to provide tenderness or protection, I endured many occasions of Mum's violence, as well as sexual abuse by two paedophiles. There was no safety in childhood. It makes sense that I now experience a complex, confusing combination of 'I love you and I hate you' and 'come here, go away' in my relationship with Michael. I become nasty when I think he might abandon me and yet my terrible behaviour will most certainly push him to leave me. Realising that my hurtful behaviour stems from childhood trauma helps me approach my relationship with Michael with greater understanding and care.

In this way, I begin the slow process of learning to love with intent. I buy a small book that still sits on my bookshelf thirty years later, *When Anger Hurts Your Relationship* by Matthew McKay and Kim Paleg. Following every suggested step, I gradually learn to breathe through my anger, to walk away instead of saying the cruel words that form themselves in my head unbidden. Determined not to be like Mum, I don't hit, yell, throw things or slam doors. Tiny step by tiny step, I realise I need not allow my childhood trauma to poison the growing bond between Michael and me.

Understanding my triggers allows me to regulate my emotions, giving rise to a growing sense of self-kindness. My childhood doesn't define me and my past need no longer predict my future. I learn to resolve conflict without ugly fights and discover that it's safe to be vulnerable with Michael. In the process, I heal from past traumas. Over the decades that follow, Michael and I steadily tend the safety and respect of our loving bond.

CHAPTER TWO

1993-1999

Having graduated from university, I'm studying a master's degree in couple and family therapy and have a job in Darlinghurst, providing individual and group therapy to young people who have experienced suicidal ideation or attempted suicide. It's a privilege to assist my young clients on their journeys of healing, just as Robbie helped me on my own. Most clients attending our service have experienced traumatic childhoods, including domestic violence and sexual abuse, with interpersonal trauma being one of the key predictors of suicidal impulses. My childhood experiences now provide me with a kind of superpower – the power of having faced my own suffering and of painstakingly built a life of purpose. Holding hope for my clients during their time of suffering is a task I gratefully embrace.

Returning to the Taoist wisdom that each life is made of ten thousand joys and ten thousand sorrows, I recognise that I'm finally being graced with the joys – among them, the profound privilege of sharing hope and compassion with others. Over time, I grow into a valued part of the team – with colleagues who become trusted friends. Surrounded by a circle of women who uplift me with their laughter, support and care, I feel a sense of wholeness I've never known before. The days of sex work and dependence on the former guru are in the distant past. How grateful I am for this stability and kindness. I've stopped believing the old stories – that I'm too flawed, too messed up, too big, or simply too much.

158

§

Michael and I marry in 1995. The biggest surprise of all is that, despite having vowed not to have children, I suddenly discover within me a profound yearning to have a child in my mid-thirties. Could it be the ticking of my biological clock, or is it the deep sense of safety in our marriage that's awakened this desire for a child? Michael and I endlessly discuss the topic of becoming parents. What kind of parents do we want to be? How will we be different to our own parents? What will our baby look like? What will we name our child? Soon, I have expensive microsurgery to have my sterilisation reversed. We're going to be parents and our lives are full of promise.

§

Still not pregnant eighteen months later, I find myself lying on a gynae-cologist's couch at the Royal Women's Hospital, my legs in stirrups and Doctor Jeffrey's head between them. As I undergo a dye test of my tubes, I hold my breath and cross my fingers. *May my fallopian tubes be ready for pregnancy*, I pray. *May they be healthy and robust.*

'Your fallopian tubes have closed over again. You'll never have a baby,' Doctor Jeffrey tells me as he washes his hands. His voice is brisk and indifferent.

I start to sob.

'You've got mascara all over your face,' he says, scribbling something in his notes. He doesn't tell me there are other options, such as IVF, doesn't pass me a box of tissues, doesn't give me hope. I can hear the unspoken words he doesn't say: You only have yourself to blame. I agree with Doctor Jeffrey; it's all my fault.

As I walk out of the gynaecologist's room, I sob loudly. Michael steps out of the waiting room and wraps me in his arms. He rubs my back in circles as I weep. I know I'm being punished for the reckless decision I made at twenty-five, for following the guru's command that all his devotees should be sterilised. I think back to the ashram in America, where not a single child was born during the four years of its existence. What a fool I was to follow the gurus' orders.

After Doctor Jeffrey's prognosis, I experience months of profound remorse. Of all the harm I've endured in my devotion to the guru, this injury cuts the deepest. Deeper than the sex work, deeper than digging ditches twelve hours a day and sleeping in a tiny space with two roommates. Michael and I stop trying for a baby, and I return to Robbie to deal with my grief.

§

A few months later I suffer days of nausea. In the middle of the night, I discover an old pregnancy test in the back of a bathroom drawer. I pee on the stick, just in case. The result is positive. My heart pounds rapidly inside my chest. At four in the morning, unable to wait any longer, I drive through the dark to the all-night chemist in Kings Cross and buy two more pregnancy tests. I come home, my hands shaking, and take them again. Both are positive – a miracle has just occurred. Jumping up and down on our bed, I wake Michael.

'I'm pregnant! You're gonna be a dad,' I yell.

Michael and I walk around in a state of rapture. We're going to be parents and are smitten with our baby already. We lie in bed, holding hands and calling out baby names. We giggle wildly and abundantly. We feel like we are the first pregnant couple on this wonderful planet.

§

Some weeks later though, I hang over the gutter on Victoria Street in Darlinghurst on my way to work. I vomit up the breakfast I forced myself to eat: dry toast with a smear of Vegemite and no butter, and a cup of ginger tea for the nausea. The sun is too bright against my closed eyelids as people walk past and create as much distance as they can from me. They probably think I'm drunk. I'm thirty-eight years old and four months pregnant. Although I've longed intensely for this pregnancy, I'm lost in a sea of misery. Vomit splashes onto my new clogs and tears stream down my face. My excitement has vanished, replaced by fear. I'm scared of the baby and am convinced I'll be a terrible mum.

Instead of going to work, I drive to the Women's Hospital in Randwick. Crying, I walk into the emergency department where a midwife with red curls and freckles gently steers me into one of the consulting rooms. The room is cold and clinical, but her manner is reassuring. She's wearing pink scrubs with smiling panda bears and she looks at me warmly.

'I'm Wendy, tell me what's going on.' Her voice and attentive green eyes show care.

'I'm four months pregnant and I'm vomiting day and night. I can't keep anything down. I thought the morning sickness would be over after three months. Also, I have a history of childhood abuse and I'm scared I'll hurt my baby after it's born.' My hands shake and intense nausea consumes me.

I tell Wendy that I shouldn't be a mum and that Children's Services will take my baby away, because I'm certain I'll harm it.

'Okay, let's deal with one issue at a time. Firstly, you have what's called hyperemesis, the term for constant vomiting. It's a major predictor of perinatal depression. Also, your baby won't be able to grow properly if you're not keeping anything down. We're going to get you admitted and put in a drip, so you can be properly hydrated.

I promise you'll feel so much better with some fluids inside you. We'll keep you in hospital for a day or two.' Wendy smiles reassuringly.

I'm grateful there are people who can help me.

'I'll call Doctor Bartley, our psychiatrist. She'll do an assessment and take on your care during your pregnancy. I'm sure you'll be a good mum, Martina. Try not to believe your negative thoughts,' she tells me.

If only I could.

Wendy walks me to the ward, her shoes squeaking on the green lino floors. She shows me to my bed and I change into a blue gown that ties at the back. I lie down on a slippery plastic mattress covered by a thin white sheet. There are three large-bellied women in the other beds. They laugh and chat, and I just know they'll be great mums. And here I am, filled with fear that I'll end up hurting the very child I want to love and protect.

The visions of violence are so extreme I can't tell anyone about them. I'm certain I'll punch and slap my baby, that I might put my hands around her tiny neck and squeeze, or cause purple bruises on her tiny squishy arms. The visions are terrifying, and I can't stop them marching through my brain like an army of soldiers trained to torture. Hot shame trickles down my armpits – about being sexually abused, about being a former sex worker, about having PTSD, and most of all, about not bonding with the baby inside me. All the women on this ward know what they're doing, while I'm already a bad and dangerous mother. Even though my baby is merely the size of an avocado, I worry that my dark thoughts are already causing it harm. Wendy covers me with a white waffle blanket and hands me a green plastic dish to vomit into. She finds a vein in my left hand and attaches a bag of saline to a metal stand.

'The IV therapy will help replace lost electrolytes. It contains

minerals and vitamins to offer you and the baby nutritional support.'
She gives me some tablets for the nausea and a glass of water.

'You should feel a lot better in an hour or two.' Wendy squeezes
my shoulder.

After a couple of hours, a tall woman with a plump body
signalling comfort walks into the ward. She has grey hair and thick
purple glasses.

'I'm Doctor Bartley, the Perinatal Psychiatrist.' She shakes my
hand. 'Please call me Hannah.'

She pulls the pale-yellow curtains closed around me and I
already feel a little safer. This woman will help me, she looks
capable, and I instinctively sense that she cares. A seed of hope
plants itself inside my dark heart. Doctor Bartley pulls up a chair
and asks me questions about my childhood and nods as I tell her
about the sexual abuse and complex post-traumatic stress diagnosis.

'I'm scared I'll hurt the baby,' I whisper, avoiding eye contact.

'Do you have a pet?' she asks me.

'Yes, I have a dog and a cat.'

'Do you feed them regularly?' she asks.

'Twice a day.'

'Do you ever punish them, hit them?'

'Of course not,' I reply, feeling a little offended.

'Usually, people who abuse their children also mistreat their
animals because both are vulnerable and dependent,' she explains,
smiling at me.

It can't be that simple.

'I'd never harm my pets. But I *will* harm my baby,' I insist, still
avoiding eye contact.

We continue to talk for nearly an hour.

'I'd like to see you weekly until baby arrives. Then we'll book you
in for an inpatient stay at our Mother-and-Baby Unit once you've

163

given birth, so we can keep an eye on you both. We'll help you form a secure bond with baby. I'm certain you'll be a lovely mum. We'll make sure your experiences in childhood don't repeat themselves.' She looks at me with such confidence that I nearly believe her.

'You have what's called perinatal psychosis, stemming from your childhood trauma. About one in a thousand women experience psychosis during pregnancy. This is what is causing your delusions and creating obsessive, false beliefs about yourself. The onset of psychosis is an emergency and it's important that you receive immediate help. It's not your fault and you're not to blame. We'll get you through this, Martina.' Doctor Bartley's voice is calm and reassuring.

'Thank you,' I whisper, relief flooding my body.

'We'll give you some medication to help with your overwhelming thoughts. You'll have weekly therapy sessions with me until you no longer need my support.' Doctor Bartley gently touches my shoulder.

I'm relieved there's a name for this hell: perinatal psychosis. If other women also experience this, maybe I'm not a monster after all.

When she leaves, I lie on the hospital bed and focus on my breathing. Placing my hand on my belly, I connect for the first time with the baby growing inside me.

'Hi baby, I'm gonna try to be a good mum,' I whisper as I rub my belly in circles.

Over the months of my pregnancy, I work hard to dispel the negative beliefs I harbour about becoming a mother. I attend weekly appointments with Doctor Bartley and have therapy sessions with Robbie once a month. Coming to understand that my past doesn't predict my future, I slowly realise I have the power to intentionally become a better mother than my own. Even though she inflicted violence in childhood, I have a choice about how I will care for our baby. During this time, I'm called to grieve my childhood once again, allowing me to become a conscious and loving mum to our baby. My mother-wound is as painful as the sexual abuse.

In therapy, I realise that my brothers and I received no tenderness from Mum because she was depressed and suicidal, with an unsupportive husband and three children under five. Mum meted out harsh physical punishments, but even more harmful was the lack of simple kindness and predictability in our home. While Mum cleaned, polished, cooked and made our beds with hospital corners, something essential was missing in our home. We were unsafe and unloved because Mum had been unsafe and unloved in her childhood. Little by little, I begin to trust that I can be a different, better mum than my own, and I feel deeply grateful to be walking this sacred path of healing.

§

On the night I go into labour, Michael and I are in the middle of a fight. I don't remember what it was about. We get into bed, furious with each other. We lie with our sides turned away from one another, as far apart as our queen-sized bed will allow. My large belly almost hangs off the mattress. The full moon outside the bedroom window shines onto our unhappy bed. Michael pulls the doona off me, and I angrily snatch it back.

'Goodnight,' I say, trying to soften my voice. I don't like it when we go to sleep cross with each other.

Michael doesn't reply.

'Goodnight!' I say, louder this time. My voice has quickly become angry once again.

There's no reply because he's fallen asleep. *How do men manage to fall sleep in the middle of an argument?* I wonder. I lie in bed and fume. My belly is huge and I can't get comfortable. Suddenly, there is a stabbing pain down low in my stomach. Shocked, I moan with the force of it. I rub my belly in circles, trying to soothe the sharp pain that returns every few minutes. Each time it passes, I wonder whether I imagined it because there's no hint of pain between the contractions. It's three weeks before my due date, so this shouldn't be happening yet. I only just started my maternity leave two days ago.

An hour later, I wake Michael.

'The baby's coming! I'm having contractions; can you run me a bath?' I yell excitedly.

He jumps out of bed and runs a bath.

'I've put Epsom salts and lavender in it.' Michael hugs me, smiling from ear to ear.

Our anger is gone. We giggle excitedly.

I climb into the hot bath and allow the lavender to soothe me. Later, Michael holds my hands to hoist me out of the bath. While he towels me dry, I'm suddenly thrilled and hopeful. I'll be a good mum, I won't hurt our baby and I'll know how to love it.

§

Thirty hours later, I push Lucie into the world, and the midwife places her in my arms. Her body is slippery, and her hands do a delicate dance, waving gently in the air. Her lips are pursed, ready to feed. Lucie means 'bringer of light', and here she is, shining her bright light, piercing our hearts like an arrow. I hold her on my chest while the doctor stitches me up – thirty-six stitches – in layers. I say a prayer of thanks for modern medicine and for epidurals, and I don't care about the state of my vagina because I'm in the middle of falling in love.

After months of torment that I might harm my baby, I know with certainty I'll never hurt this delicate human. I'll never lay a hand on her in anger, I will not abuse her, and I won't need an inpatient stay at the Mother-and-Baby Unit. I won't be a monster. Instead I'll get to know our baby intimately and memorise her various cries, knowing when she is hungry, tired or in pain, and I'll learn how to comfort her and meet her every need.

Michael holds Lucie as tears of joy stream down his face, his eyes red with exhaustion. He bends and kisses me, and he kisses our daughter's forehead, cheeks and hands.

'Thank you,' he says through tears. 'This is the happiest day of my life.'

Later, we're taken to a private room where Michael and I lie together on a narrow hospital bed, with Lucie's body tucked like a parcel between us. We kiss her over and over while she gazes calmly at the bedside light and continues to wave her hands. Her head turns towards me, and her mouth reaches for my breast. This is how we learn together to nourish her body and soul.

§

Michael and I bring Lucie home and delight in her expressive face, intense blue-eyed gaze, dancing hands and perfectly formed body. We're enchanted by the little noises she makes, as well as by her urgent cries and greedy gulps when she drinks at my breast. She sleeps in our bed, and on our daily walks in Centennial Park, Lucie's body is close to my heart in her baby sling, while Basil walks proudly ahead, wagging his black tail. When bathing her at the end of each day, she kicks her legs and arms in the warm water, making delighted noises.

I'm deeply grateful that at thirty-eight, and despite childhood trauma and sterilisation in my twenties, I am a good mum, neither abusive nor crazy. Lucie is our miracle.

Being a mum gives me the opportunity to care consistently for a vulnerable human being. Loving Lucie heals me as much as the years of therapy with Robbie. By giving our baby the care I didn't experience in childhood, I too receive love. Every time I show Lucie tenderness, I experience healing. She is a happy baby who giggles loudly when she pulls Basil's ears and tail. She screams with delight when he licks her face with his rough pink tongue. When Lucie sleeps in her bassinet, Basil sits and guards her closely. The greatest gift of all is that Michael and I provide a home and family that is predictable and kind.

CHAPTER THREE

1999

It's early summer and Lucie is six months old. I carry her upstairs to change her nappy, her little legs wrapped around my waist, and her hands hot and sticky around my neck. I put her on our bed where she gurgles and smiles, waving her arms and legs. Overwhelmed with love, I change her nappy and gaze at her vulva. Her legs are spread, and I suddenly feel sick. How could my perpetrators have harmed me when I was just as innocent as Lucie? I nearly begin to cry, but I must keep it together for Lucie. Determined that the intergenerational family curse must stop with me, I'll not allow my trauma to be passed down to her. She doesn't need a mum like mine, screaming and threatening suicide.

I put a clean nappy on Lucie and gently tickle her. We giggle together. But while I blow a raspberry kiss on her tummy, I feel the insistent curse of my childhood once again. I dress Lucie in her blue-and-red-striped jumpsuit and gently put her in her cot for her afternoon nap. As I sing to her and stroke her hair, her eyes are heavy with sleep.

'Twinkle twinkle little star, how I wonder what you are,' I sing.

Kissing her face, forehead and hands, I draw the curtains and softly close the bedroom door. Lucie is a good sleeper, and I remind myself she is safe from harm.

Downstairs, I shut the door to the living room and cry quietly. Basil sits next to me, his amber eyes full of concern. I hold my face in my hands to soothe the pain of the memories. I try to calm myself by taking slow deliberate breaths like Robbie taught me. I consider my own innocence, and how Grandpa and Uncle hurt me without concern for the small, sweet girl I was.

I hear the school bell ring. It's three in the afternoon. I get up and watch the children from the local primary school across the road as they yell, jump, run and laugh, their voices a joyous song. They wear maroon and yellow shorts, tops and bucket hats. When their mums pick them up, the children put on their backpacks, enormous on their tiny bodies. They look like turtles standing on their hind legs. The mums hold their hands as they walk down the road. Mum never held my hand when she picked me up from school.

The phone rings. I blow my nose and pick it up. It's Mum from Switzerland.

'Hello, Martina. How is Lucie?' she asks me in Swiss German, without warmth in her voice.

'She's wonderful, Mum, such a happy baby. She's having her afternoon nap.' I try to sound normal.

'What's wrong with you? You sound strange.' Mum is an expert at reading my moods.

'I'm just feeling sad about the sexual abuse. Having Lucie has triggered some of my old memories,' I tell Mum, tears forming in my eyes.

'Oh, here we go again. It's always about you, you, you, isn't it! When are you going to stop thinking the world revolves around you?' Mum yells.

'But you're my mum. Why can't you support me?' I plead with her.

'I'm sick of you making me feel guilty. It wasn't my fault.' While she believes the abuse happened, I must never complain about it.

'But why can't you be compassionate towards me? You're my mum,' I beg.

'Oh, for God's sake, stop this self-pity,' Mum hisses.

I begin to wail, and she hangs up on me – a loud click, then silence at the end of the line. Curling up on the blue couch in the foetal position, my tears drip onto the pillow. I don't have the energy to get the tissues. Thank God Lucie's upstairs asleep and can't see me cry. Mum always manages to break my heart. Maybe I should stop having contact with her. She always makes me feel worse.

Michael comes into the lounge room, home from work.

'What's wrong?' He hugs me as I sob into his shoulder.

'Mum rang. She told me to stop talking about the abuse. She says I'm selfish,' I cry.

Michael brings me tissues and a cup of tea. He holds my hands and strokes my hair.

'You're not selfish. That's it, I'm ringing her,' he says.

He picks up the phone and rings Mum in Switzerland, fifteen buttons on the dial. She picks up the phone.

'Susanne, it's Michael,' he says. 'We need to talk about Martina. She's very distressed. You've really hurt her, and I want you to apologise to her,' Michael says firmly.

I hear Mum yell for a long time while Michael listens patiently.

'No, Susanne, you must apologise to Martina. I want you to do it right now.' His voice is resolute.

I can't believe he's talking to Mum like this. No one ever dares challenge her, not even Dad. Suddenly elated, I'm filled with gratitude at Michael's courage and kindness. The little girl within me is exhilarated. Michael is not afraid of Mum.

He hands me the phone.

'Sorry!' Mum sounds resentful.

She clearly doesn't mean it and is only saying sorry because Michael told her to. Though I know her apology isn't genuine, it sends a thrill through me.

'Thank you, Mum,' I say, smiling. I hang up, feeling ecstatic. This is the very first sorry I've ever received from Mum.

Michael and I hug and laugh at the miracle of her begrudging apology.

I go to the bathroom and wash my face. As I look at my reflection in the mirror, I remind myself I am a strong adult. Robbie has taught me well. Glad to be her safe haven, I smile knowing Lucie will always be cherished.

Soon I hear Lucie call out from her cot, 'Mammmammmamum.'

I pick her up and give her loud kisses as she giggles into my neck. Joy courses between our bodies. Downstairs we sit on the sofa, where a short time ago I cried inconsolably. I pull up my top and Lucie begins to suckle noisily while she pats my breast with her chubby hand. She looks up at me with complete trust, and I gaze back at her – such endless love.

'I love you, my darling.' I smile as she continues to pat me.

CHAPTER FOUR

2003

Michael, Lucie and I have left Sydney and now live on a property on the mid-north coast of New South Wales. Lucie goes to the local daycare, Michael works as a welfare worker at the primary school, and I've taken a job with the government Sexual Assault Service in Taree.

Mum and Dad are visiting from Switzerland and staying with us for three days, the maximum amount of time I'm able to tolerate them. Michael, Lucie and Dad have gone to the beach for a swim, and Mum and I have decided to stay back at the house. We sit on the veranda and look out at the dry summer bush, the ancient sound of cicadas a thrumming pulse all around us. A wallaby mum and her joey graze nearby.

Mum and I smile. We rarely smile together, so I enjoy this moment. We speak quietly so we don't startle the wallabies. Soon, the joey makes its way back to its mum's pouch while the mum continues to graze on the dry brown grass and scan for danger.

'I want to tell you about my childhood,' Mum says.

She tells me that she recently discovered that her father has a Wikipedia page with all the articles he wrote when he was a celebrated judge and scholar.

'I threw out all the books he published, but now he's on the damn internet.' Mum sighs.

I've heard this story a few times, and though I instinctively brace myself for the familiar litany, I choose to be patient with her.

'On the internet, it doesn't say he was a criminal,' she's shouting now.

She tells me he was a dictator in the courtroom and at home, where he ruled with a loud voice and violent fists. Even when he became bedridden after his stroke, he remained frightening. Mum's voice continues to rise with hurt and anger and the wallaby hops away, disappearing into the bush.

'It must have been terrible growing up with your father,' I say. I try to show empathy, but I push my legs and feet into the floor of the veranda to contain my impatience.

'No one protected me, not even my own mother,' Mum replies.

I remember well from my own childhood that Grandma was her husband's handmaiden. Her *raison d'être* was to serve him and her son. She was cruel to Mum, her only daughter, and neglected her. Grandma didn't protect Mum from her father and brother's abuse.

'Men and boys were everything and girls were worthless.' Tears run down Mum's cheeks. 'I hated my brother too.'

I go inside and fetch a box of tissues for Mum. I think about Grandma, the way she passed her internalised misogyny on to Mum, who handed it down to me, like a baton in a relay race. I offer Mum the tissues while wondering with some bitterness why she didn't protect me from the father and brother she hated so much. But I don't say this, because I don't want to disturb this rare moment of closeness between us. Also, if I'm honest, I continue to fear her anger.

I remember how Grandma always cooked my favourite meals and took me to the supermarket with her, where I got to choose sweet treats including ice cream and chocolate. Our times at the supermarket were special.

'Grandma loved me, but she didn't protect me either.' I pick at my cuticles and my middle finger begins to throb.

'She was much nicer to you than she was to me.' Mum's face has hardened with resentment.

She continues to talk about her childhood, saying her brother also has a Wikipedia page that doesn't mention he was a paedophile. He craved public adoration and, as a popular politician, he regularly appeared on television to discuss current affairs.

'I remember one night when I was about seven, we watched the evening news. Suddenly, Uncle appeared on the TV screen, and I ran to the bathroom and hid.' I continue to pick at my cuticles. 'I thought he had come to our house through the television set and that he was going to hurt me. ' I dig my nails into the palms of my hands.

'I don't remember that,' Mum says dismissively. 'He gave talks about social justice and women's rights. What a hypocrite!' She is shouting again – the wallabies are long gone.

I think about Uncle and how he disguised the monster inside by casting a convincing light. Everyone was drawn to his surface charm – including me. I loved him once, fooled by his charisma and humour, unaware it was part of his grooming process.

'Do you think your dad and brother sexually abused you too, Mum?' I ask.

'I'm quite sure they did, and I do have some vague memories.' Her face is set in a painful grimace.

I reflect about Mum's hatred of them, her threats of suicide, the powerful rages and profound despair – all possible signs of trauma from sexual abuse, according to psychological research.

'Mum, you also had the same bladder problems I always had. That may be a sign of abuse,' I say, my thighs and toes tightly clenched.

Mum and I both suffered from urinary tract infections, and we had to bathe with purple Condy's Crystals to soothe our pain.

'I remember one day I visited my parents when I was in my mid-thirties, your grandpa shouted at me, and I was so scared I wet my pants,' Mum reflects.

I remember this day too. Mum ran out of the house and just left me there with the perpetrators.

'I sobbed all the way home,' Mum says.

'I'm sorry you were so scared of him,' I reply briskly, biting the inside of my cheek.

But why did you leave me with your father if you were so terrified of him? I think bitterly. But I say nothing. Mum still has more power than I do.

'I was very smart at school, and my dream was to become a doctor,' Mum ponders.

Instead, her parents pulled her out of school at fifteen and put her in nursing college in Zurich. She loved being a nurse in another city, far away from her loveless family.

I remember her telling me that with every monthly pay, she bought new shoes – her favourite purchase. She had a collection of a dozen shoes and felt elegant in her heels as she walked beside Lake Zurich with her nursing friends, laughing and carefree.

'I worked as a nurse until I married your father. In 1950s Switzerland, married women were confined to the home and weren't allowed to keep working.' Mum blows her nose and dabs at her face.

'That's so unfair. You loved earning your own money and being free,' I say.

Mum tells me she always came second best to her brother, who was given tennis lessons, private maths coaching, expensive overseas holidays and designer shoes and clothes.

'When I grew breasts at fourteen, Mum told me she couldn't afford to buy me a bra. Instead, she gave me one of her grimy old ones that didn't even fit me properly.' Mum is shredding a wad of tissues.

In her teens, every summer her parents and brother went on a month's seaside holiday in Italy, leaving her at home on her own. Every day, a kind neighbour looked in on her and dropped off a hot meal.

'You must have felt so hurt, Mum.' I want to touch her, but we don't touch in our family.

We continue to sit side by side, not looking at each other. Feeling conflicted, I have empathy for her suffering on one hand, and anger on the other. Why didn't she keep me safe?

'I always rang my mother twice a week after I left home. I still wanted her to love me,' Mum says bitterly.

I nod in sympathy. I understand firsthand the enduring longing for a different, more loving mother.

'Mum, if you'd been born in the sixties, you could have studied medicine, become a doctor and kept working after you got married.' I gnaw at my nails.

Mum doesn't reply. She blows her nose again and wipes her face with a tissue.

I remember being in the living room in my playpen and observing Mum through the wooden bars. As a toddler, I already knew she was unhappy, and could sense her every mood – I always tried extra hard to make her smile.

As we sit together on the veranda, I continue to reflect that Mum and I had many things in common, including insomnia, anxiety, depression, fear of and anger at men, addiction to pills, body shame and disordered eating. I glance at Mum who is continuing to shred her tissues.

I also remember that when Mum was with her nursing friends, she became a vibrant, joyful woman. I loved seeing her with her girlfriends. One day I hid behind the white sofa in the living room to eavesdrop on her phone conversation with her best friend, Roni. As I peeked out, she laughed loudly with her mouth wide open. I was intoxicated by this woman who was more than my mum, and I basked in her happiness.

Having held tightly onto my anger towards Mum for decades, I now experience a moment of inner softening as we sit side by side. While there will always be some hurt and resentment, I've been able to build a life of stability and kindness. I am a loving and predictable mum, and this is the ultimate gift of my hard-won healing.

§

I watch Michael's car come up the dirt drive, and soon Lucie, Michael, Dad and Basil pile out. Mum walks over to them, and Lucie runs to me, sits on my lap in her wet swimmers and wraps her sandy arms and legs around me. She smells of sunscreen.

'I don't like Grandma. She told me my cheeks are fat. She's a mean lady,' Lucie whispers in my ear.

I give her loud kisses on her face and hands. 'You're absolute perfection, my darling, exactly the way you are. Your cheeks are so delicious I'm going to eat them.' Lucie giggles.

Later, I take Mum aside. 'Please don't say anything to Lucie about having fat cheeks. I'm teaching her body positivity, and we don't allow fat phobia in this house,' I say firmly.

Mum shrugs and walks out of the room without a word.

While there's peace between us now, I've accepted that I'll never have the mother I once longed for. And that's okay. I've found my own steadiness with which I mother Lucie, and even myself, with enduring patience and kindness. The promise of ten thousand joys has finally been fulfilled.

CHAPTER FIVE

2006

Seven-year-old Lucie and I are lying on the queen-sized bed, reading *The Bipolar Bear Family* together, a story written by Angela Ann Holloway about a young bear cub who struggles to understand his mum's bipolar disorder. An enormous, orange full moon shines through the large glass sliding door, flooding golden light onto our bed, while the frogs in the dam call out a joyful cacophony.

Inside the bedroom, I try to help Lucie understand her dad's illness. Michael was diagnosed three weeks ago with bipolar disorder and is having an inpatient stay in a psychiatric hospital two hours' drive away. As we turn the pages of the book, we pause and chat.

'Is it my fault?' Lucie asks.

'No, Lucie, Dad's illness is nobody's fault.' I stroke her forehead.

'But how long will he be in hospital?' Lucie's lip trembles.

'We're not sure yet how long. I know you miss him, and he misses you lots too.' I continue to stroke her forehead.

I tell her it will take time for the medicine to work and that he is also having a treatment called ECT.

'What's ECT, Mama?' Lucie looks scared.

'It helps people when they're very sad.' I stroke her cheek.

I don't want her to suffer.

'But why is Dad sad?' Lucie's voice is shaky.

'Sadness is part of his illness,' I explain. I hold her hand and gently squeeze it.

'Will I be a polar bear too?'

'No, you're healthy and well,' I reassure her.

I speak with confidence, but inside, I'm shaking with a fear I can't show – aware that thirty per cent of people with bipolar attempt suicide, and twenty per cent don't survive. As a psychotherapist, I know how serious such plans are. I deliberately slow and deepen my breath so that Lucie doesn't pick up my fear.

'Will Dad be a polar bear forever?' Lucie asks.

'The illness will come and go, but he'll be well most of the time. His doctor Alan specialises in helping people with bipolar.'

'Can I write the doctor a letter?'

'Of course.'

Lucie gets out of bed and fetches some paper and a pencil. Her handwriting scratches across the page:

> Dear Dokta Allen,
> thank you for luking after my dad. Pleese make him well again. Thank you from Lucie.

I turn out the light, and we settle into our pillows, holding hands.

'Mama, I can smell Dad,' she says contentedly, nestled on his side of the bed, her head resting on his pillow.

§

The next day, I drop Lucie at school and drive to Newcastle to visit Michael. My stomach tightens the closer I get to the hospital. A heavy stone has made a home inside my body. I dread seeing Michael so transformed. My husband, once full of happiness, now carries a vacant look in his eyes, his face a silent mask.

His psychiatrist explained last week that because Michael has

180

treatment-resistant depression, the typical antidepressants aren't effective. ECT will provide faster relief than the new antidepressants he's trialling. We need hope, and soon.

As I walk through the entrance of the hospital, I'm hit by the ammonia smell common to all hospitals. I knock on Michael's door.

'Come in,' he calls out, and I open the door.

He's sitting in an armchair, wearing a navy hoodie and track pants, his face grey and his facial expression flat. He stands up, smiles, and we hug. The room has a single bed, an armchair and a small white basin. My heart sinks. I don't know how Michael will get well in this sterile room. I remind myself to bring him a colourful doona next time I visit, to remind him he has a home, a family, and there is hope.

I give him a block of his favourite Lindt chocolate, and we lie on our backs on his bed, on top of his white hospital blanket. Feeling its waffle weave through my summer dress, we hold hands and share the chocolate. We devour the whole block because we need sweetness. Tears silently trickle down the sides of my face and pool in my ears. I want Michael to keep looking straight ahead, so he doesn't see me cry.

'Are you feeling suicidal?' I ask.

'A little.'

He tries to protect me, and I know he hardly ever tells me the whole truth about his illness.

'Have you got a plan?'

'I don't have one here, because they watch me all the time,' he says sadly.

I look out the window at the grey corrugated iron fence as we continue to hold hands.

'What's ECT like?' I ask.

He tells me how he lies down on a gurney in a hospital gown three mornings a week and that he can't eat or drink beforehand.

'I'm a piece of meat lying there. They give me a general anaesthetic and put paddles on my head to make me have a seizure.' Michael sounds so sad.

He tells me that when he wakes up, he's confused and has a headache for the rest of the day.

'You're brave,' I say, squeezing his hand.

We turn our bodies towards one another and look into each other's eyes.

I exhale. I've read everything I can find on ECT. Some articles say it's a barbaric, outdated practice; others say it saves lives. I don't know how we'll navigate this illness long term. But I don't tell him what I'm thinking.

'Do you want to leave me? I wouldn't blame you,' Michael says.

'No, I'm not leaving you, lovey.' I rub my thumb over the back of his hand.

'I don't want to be a burden,' he replies.

I watch his stomach rise and fall. He's alive. Please stay alive.

'Remember how unwell I was when I was pregnant? You were there for me, so I'm going to be here for you too,' I tell him.

We continue to lie on the narrow hospital bed together, our heads on the thinly covered plastic pillow that makes a crinkling noise each time we move. We have no answers, but we have love.

§

2012

Six years later, I'm in the car outside work at Newcastle Sexual Assault Service. We've recently moved to Newcastle for Lucie's high school and because I'm doing a PhD at Newcastle university. In the car, I dial Michael's mobile number for the twentieth time. I hear the whoosh of cars driving past as I weep behind the car's tinted windows. I fear Michael has finally managed to kill himself. Shaking all over, I dial his number again. He's not picking up. He always picks up! My stomach drops; it's filled with the acid of terror.

Michael is in hospital with his second bout of bipolar illness. Michael's depression is relentless, and it tells him to kill himself dozens of times every hour. That's why he's being cared for in the hospital, where he's safe from harm. I dial the hospital and ask to be put through to the nurses' station.

'Hi, it's Martina here, Michael's wife. I've been ringing Michael, but he's not picking up, which is not like him. I'm just wondering whether you've seen him.' My voice is shaky and small.

'I gave him his morning medication about two hours ago. I haven't seen him since then,' the nurse replies.

'Could you please go and have a look for him? I'm a bit worried.'

'Okay, I'll find him and get him to call you.'

Terrified, I wait for his call. I wait and I wait. I dial his number a few more times. Each time, I get his voicemail. My hands and feet are freezing cold. I can't go back into work. My husband could be dead and I don't know what to do, other than sit in the bubble of my car, aghast. How will I tell Lucie? How will we manage financially? Where are all the PIN numbers? How do I organise a funeral? How will Lucie cope without her dad? They have such a close bond. She'll have to go to after-school care. My thoughts somersault inside my head. Lucie is twelve and going through a complicated early adolescence. She is often grumpy and unkind, and I'm terrified of dealing with a sullen adolescent on my own. I pray that Michael is alive.

I call our receptionist at work.

'Maria, I've just gone to a doctor's appointment. I should be back in a couple of hours,' I say, trying to sound normal.

'Okay, love, see you soon,' she replies in her sunny voice, just living an ordinary day.

I'm so scared I can't bear it. It's as though there are ants crawling under my skin. The hospital has a duty of care; they can't just lose him. I call the nurses' station again.

'Just wondering whether you've found Michael yet?' I ask, my voice shaking.

'We're still looking for him, Martina. We'll call you as soon as we find him.' I detect a note of fear in her voice, too.

Inside the car, I whimper. My body is a giant heartbeat pulsating loudly. 'Michael, Michael, Michael, where are you? Don't do this to us,' I beg.

The phone rings and I answer it.

'Hi, darling,' Michael says.

'Where the fuck have you been? I've been so worried. They've been looking for you everywhere. I thought you were dead.' The words tumble out, equal parts relief and anger.

'I've been in the group room listening to music with my headphones on. The phone was switched off,' Michael explains. 'I'm sorry you were worried.'

'You can't just switch your phone off. I have to know whether you're alive!' I yell. I'm angry, but terror cowers just a hair's breadth beneath.

'I'm really sorry I scared you,' Michael says again.

'It's okay.' I sound surly. I should be kind to him. After all, he's the one who is sick. *I'm such a bitch*. I berate myself.

'I love you, but I'm really scared,' I say, exhausted.

I lower the driver's seat, lie back and close my eyes.

'I know. I hate bipolar. I don't recognise myself,' he replies sadly.

'Please don't die. Lucie and I need you.' I rub my temples. A headache has taken hold inside my head.

'I won't do that to Lucie or you.' He sounds so tired.

We remain silent for a couple of minutes. There's nothing to say.

I sit back up and look in the rear-view mirror and use a tissue to wipe streaks of mascara from my face, flooded with relief that Michael is alive. We say goodbye, and I climb out of the car and walk across the road. Opening the heavy glass door of the old hospital building, I slowly make my way up the stairs and back to work. My knees shake, and my head is pounding.

§

2020

I've been reading research that states eighty per cent of marriages fail when one partner suffers with bipolar disorder. I understand this. Living with Michael's illness has been hard for all of us, and I'm grateful we haven't become a statistic.

Tonight, I decide to share with Michael the chapter I've written about his illness. He's given me his blessing to write it, but I've hesitated to show him, afraid it might stir up old pain. He's been stable for several years, continues to be on a regime of medications, and regularly attends counselling. Bipolar disorder is a lifelong condition. He's in remission, but there are no certainties.

Michael and I are still in Newcastle, while Lucie lives in Sydney where she's studying at university. We're sitting at the dining room table and have just finished eating grilled salmon and salad for dinner. Reggie, our labradoodle, hovers at our feet, watching intently and hoping for some leftovers. I'm not sure how Michael will feel reading about Lucie's and my experiences of his illness. I don't want my words to hurt him, but being open and brave has always been part of how we love each other.

As he begins to read the chapter, time stands still. While I hold my breath and watch his face, I pick at my cuticles under the table. My thumb starts to bleed. I wrap a paper serviette around it to stem the blood. As I try to read Michael's facial expression, he looks intently at the computer screen. It seems to take him forever to read the chapter, while I continue to hold my breath. I watch his tears flow. He uses his serviette to wipe them away.

'Thank you for writing this,' he tells me. He reaches for my hand, and I put my head on his shoulder. 'I'd forgotten a lot of this.' We look out the window, holding hands.

'And yet, after thirty years, we're still here together.' I smile.

I remind him that his illness has been much harder on him than on me and that I'm sorry I've sometimes seemed distant and even cold towards him.

'It's because I was so scared I'd lose you,' I say.

We continue to sit at the dining table, holding hands, sensing into all the ups and downs of our marriage. The mood between us is peaceful. How did we learn to choose love, again and again, despite my dysfunctional childhood, Michael's illness and my trouble liking – let alone trusting – men?

'Do you think I should send Lucie the chapter?' I ask Michael.

'Yes, she'll want to read it.'

I worry she'll be upset, but we've always been open with her, and this is an important part of our family's story. Love and honesty have carried us through so much.

Michael clears the dishes and puts some salmon in Reggie's bowl. Reggie gobbles it up while I email Lucie the chapter about her dad's illness.

'I've sent you a chapter to read. Let me know your thoughts,' I text Lucie.

§

'Is there anything you remember that you would like me to add to make the story more authentic? Or is there anything you want me to take out? I'd love to include all our perspectives,' I write in my email to Lucie.

She rings me an hour later, her voice full of emotion.

'I remember you told Dad we were going to move out if he didn't get help,' she tells me.

I'd forgotten that we'd looked at a place to rent near her primary school when Michael was refusing to get treatment.

'He was gutted at the thought of us moving out, and that's what made him finally agree to get help,' Lucie reminds me.

'Yes, the next day he was admitted to hospital. I'm so glad things are good for Dad now,' I tell her, awed at the journey we've been through.

I take the phone into the bedroom and lie on the bed in the dark as we continue to remember together.

She tells me that the hardest part for her was hearing me say that her dad would be home in a couple of weeks – until those weeks stretched into three long months.

'You weren't honest about how long he'd be gone until I was much older, in high school.' Lucie's voice is sad.

'You're right, I'm sorry, Lucie. That was a mistake,' I reply, feeling guilty.

'Yes, the worst part for me was that you were both not being honest with me,' she says over the phone.

'That was wrong of us. I'm very sorry,' I reply.

'I'm not angry now. You don't have to apologise; you were just trying to protect me,' Lucie says sadly.

'Thanks, Lucie. It was a really hard time for all of us, wasn't it?'

Tears trickle down the sides of my face and pool in my ears as I lie in the dark. I'm sure she's crying too.

'Another thing I remember is that one of the times when Dad was in hospital, you lost eight demerit points and got a nine-hundred -dollar driving fine in one single afternoon. Do you remember?' She giggles.

'How could I forget?' I laugh. 'I was a total mess, racing from work to get you to the dentist who booked appointments every ten minutes. You couldn't afford to be even a minute late.'

I was late, and ended up running two red lights, both times going seventy in a sixty zone. I swear they looked orange to me, but Beaumont Street's red-light camera caught me twice in less than an hour.

'Dad had to give me some of his points because I would have lost my licence,' I chuckle.

'You were crazy, Mum,' Lucie jokes.

'Yep, I really was. I was so stressed and scared.' We giggle, relieved that things are calmer now.

We chat a little longer about her honour's thesis. She'll finish university soon with a degree in social work and criminology.

'Gabe and I have bought tickets to Laos, the Philippines and Thailand.' Lucie sounds excited, and I'm grateful she's happy and embarking on new adventures.

'I'm so proud of you, darling,' I tell her.

'Thanks, Mum. I have to go. I'm going into Coles now. I love you, Mama,' she says.

'I love you lots, too, darling. Thanks for telling me about the things I could have done differently,' I say, feeling profound love for her.

After the phone call, I'm filled with gratitude. Michael is well and our daughter is safe and happy and I've been able to break the cycle of family violence.

CHAPTER SIX

2014

On a September evening, Lucie and I sit together on the red couch in the living room. I'm helping her with her history homework when the phone rings. I pick up and hear Mum's voice from Switzerland.

'Martina, your uncle died of heart failure last night.'

He never did have a heart, I think, just as an overwhelming wave of nausea hits me.

'Mum, I can't believe he's finally dead. Can I call you back in a minute?'

I hang up the phone and race upstairs. 'I'll be right back, Lucie,' I call out.

I lean over the toilet bowl, where I vomit up my dinner. Pesto pasta, salad greens with tomatoes, olives, cucumbers and blueberries – a colourful mix. Kneeling on the bathroom floor with my arms wrapped around the toilet seat, a second wave erupts and my stomach heaves. My hands shake and my body vibrates. I curl up on the floor, my forehead hot, hands and armpits clammy, sweat trickling down my back. He's finally dead. My head spins as I try to sit up, so I curl up on the floor again, dizzy and in a state of shock. There's a knock on the door.

'Mum, are you okay?' Lucie opens the door.

She's fourteen, and I want to protect her, so I sit up and try to look somewhat normal.

'What's wrong, Mum?' Lucie looks worried.

'I'll be okay, darling. Just give me a couple of minutes. Dinner didn't agree with me,' I say, panting.

When Lucie leaves, I lie on the floor, my head spinning. Eventually, I stand, wash my hands and face, rinse my mouth and look at my reflection in the mirror. I look like I've seen a ghost – my skin is a grey mask, my eyes red and watery. I look ninety years old because my uncle has taken something I can't get back.

I go into the bedroom, lie down on the bed in the dark and return Mum's call.

'Hi, Mum, I can talk now,' I say with my eyes closed.

'He's dead at last, that disgusting man. I'm so damn happy.' Mum laughs, a sound I rarely hear.

'I can't believe it, Mum. Are you going to the funeral?' I ask.

'Of course I am. I want to make sure he really is dead.' Mum's still laughing.

I can't laugh with Mum. I'm scared. I tell myself he's dead and there's nothing to fear, but an unexpected terror quakes inside my stomach. We talk for a few more minutes about the autumn in Switzerland and the trees in Mum's garden, which have turned yellow, orange and red. I can hardly hear Mum because I feel far away. Her voice sounds muffled, and my body is paralysed by an inexplicable fear.

After I hang up, I rush back to the bathroom and rid myself of Uncle's dark poison that has resided within me for half a century.

Between trips to the toilet, I tuck Lucie into her bed.

'Mum, why are you so sick?'

'Darling, Grandma rang to tell me that the uncle who abused me has just died. It's made me feel sick just thinking about him again,' I explain as I tuck her into bed.

'It's good he's dead though, isn't it, Mum?' she asks, looking worried.

'Yes, it's very good. He caused so much hurt.' I stroke her forehead.

I kiss Lucie goodnight and leave the bedroom door ajar just how she likes it.

When I climb into bed, terrifying visions of Uncle pulling me into his grave fill my mind. I'm scared I'll be buried alive with his rotting corpse – that I'll be trapped with him forever. Worms will eat my body. I toss and turn and do battle through the long night as I go back and forth to the bathroom. Reminding myself that I'm free of him at last, I find my body can't grasp the concept of his death. He has always been larger than life. Even now, his shadow lingers in the room with me – all the way from Switzerland. Like a ghost, he moves freely now that death has unshackled his body. His ghost has come to hurt me.

He never admitted the crimes he perpetrated against me, and now he never will. There will be no apology, no court case or prison sentence. No article in the newspapers listing his crimes, no television news bulletin reporting his paedophilia. I will not be vindicated. Instead, I will have to continue to find my own liber- ation. I wonder whether there will be a reckoning for him, whether there's a god who punishes paedophiles? This man, who caused so much harm, has walked away without consequence. I'm enraged by all he took from me – and that it's taken everything in me to fight the damage he inflicted. As I hang my head over the toilet bowl, I wonder how many children have suffered at his hands. In the stillness of the sleepless night, I grieve that he escaped justice, just as Grandpa did.

As the grey morning light comes through the French doors, I remind myself that I've outlived him. His body will soon be burned to ashes and fragments of bone, and he won't be able to harm any more children. I remind myself that ghosts aren't real. I'm not in his coffin with him. I'm here in Australia, a grown-up with a blessed life of love and hope. Soon I will get up, make Lucie her porridge and take her to school.

CHAPTER SEVEN

2014

After Uncle's death, old memories continue to emerge and my amygdala pings in a state of hypervigilance. I have several nightmares in short succession about the paedophiles. They are both dead, and yet they still grab at me from their graves. I remind myself that ghosts aren't real.

One morning, I sit on the couch and drink my coffee. Reggie, our labradoodle, sits beside me. I stroke his silky blonde curls while he leans into my side and groans contentedly. I place the palm of my right hand on his warm chest and feel his heartbeat.

I remind myself that my amygdala will soon settle, that the function of this tiny almond-shaped part of the brain involves experiencing emotions and memories associated with fear. I learned from Robbie that the amygdala is the brain's alarm bell, signalling immediate danger. Right now, it's like a pinball machine, pinging to keep me safe from the paedophiles, who visited me without my consent last night. I place my left hand on my heart and whisper to the small sad child that cries inside me.

'You are safe, my darling. They can't hurt you any longer. They are both dead, ashes and dust.'

'I will never be safe,' the hurt child replies as she puts her small head on my chest.

§

Robbie also taught me about the concept of the inner child in therapy. Initially, it was hard to accept my inconvenient inner child. I didn't like this needy, messy, annoying little girl. But finally, I realised that when I love and reassure her, she rewards me. So, I hold her gently on my lap and wrap my arms around her. Right now, she doesn't trust me because my amygdala is dominant and my prefrontal cortex is offline. I know from experience the prefrontal cortex will return, but it may take an hour or two.

Robbie taught me that the large prefrontal cortex located at the crown of our head, regulates our emotions and helps us reason things out. The prefrontal cortex responds more slowly than the amygdala, which is why the amygdala tends to win initially. It takes a while for the slow prefrontal cortex to bring back order, carefully assessing risk. The prefrontal cortex allows me to ask helpful questions, such as: is the danger immediate, or is it in the past? This is something I often explain to my clients in the sanctity of the therapy room. And this morning, I must heed my own advice once more as I work out there's no immediate danger.

I open my laptop and decide to write, but fear paralyses my fingers. The paedophiles tell me that I am no one and I have nothing worth saying.

'No one will believe you,' they yell from their graves.

They don't want anyone to know about the crimes they committed against the small girl I was.

I raise myself from my paralysis and take some deep breaths. I get up from the couch, open the window and stretch my body. I take in the fresh air, watch as a coal ship enters Newcastle Harbour, and look at the sparkling ocean beyond.

I am alive and I refuse to be silenced by ancestral voices.

The perpetrators keep shouting at me to 'shut the fuck up', but I refuse to obey them.

I put on my running shoes and take Reggie for his morning walk. We jog along the sparkling harbour, Reggie's tail high in the air, a joyful curly flag. Today, there are invisible landmines of trauma I must navigate. Despite decades of healing, I continue to find myself under siege at times. As an adult, I've learned to deal with my instinctive reactions to men. Yet I must manage myself daily, even on this pleasurable morning walk in the sunshine – at once healed and not healed, the ten thousand joys and sorrows colliding.

Unexpected triggers may detonate at any moment: old men, middle-aged men, bald men, men with shaved heads, men with bushy eyebrows, men with long beards, men with cleft chins, men who invade my space. Men with charming bright-blue eyes. Men who ogle my beautiful young daughter, old enough to be her father or grandfather. Men who are overly friendly.

Being alone in a lift with a man, men who unexpectedly come up behind me, jogging men breathing loudly in my vicinity, drunk men, violent men, charismatic men and, of course, judges and politicians. Men who innocently happen to sit next to me at a concert. And, obviously, paedophiles and sexual predators.

As a so-called high-functioning adult, I seemingly calmly outmanoeuvre all these potential dangers. No wonder I used pills, alcohol, cigarettes and binge eating to manage the fearful child within. Giving up these substances unexpectedly brought me the greatest freedom, yet letting go of them was terrifying at first. Without the numbness, I had to face myself – and it was excruciating. It took several tries to break free, but eventually, I did.

A man in his sixties walks towards me. He is holding the hand of a curly-haired little girl wearing red overalls. She must be about five years old. I dig my nails into the palms of my hands, my mind worrying that this man may be abusing her. Perhaps he is her grandfather. I quickly check her face, eyes and body language. Is she scared of him? Where are her parents? Is she safe?

Then I remember that my amygdala is in overdrive, that this girl is probably happy and unharmed. I remind myself I'm projecting my past onto this man and child.

Quietly, I say a small prayer for the little girl. 'May you be safe and protected, may you be happy and loved. May all children everywhere be free from harm.'

The prayer calms my body, and I continue to walk towards Nobbys Beach. Reggie sniffs the grass and cocks his leg, leaving his visiting card for other dogs.

§

Home from the walk, I sit on the couch and start typing on my laptop.

'Don't talk! Don't tell! Shut the fuck up!' The perpetrators yell once again from beyond their graves.

'Try and stop me.' I laugh in their faces, suddenly brave.

My fear has dissipated on my morning walk, and my fingers are flying across the keyboard. Each time I stand up to my ancestors' voices, I take another step towards healing. My perpetrators shall not win.

Later, I use the calculator on my phone to work out how many times the abuse occurred between 1962 and 1965. I stayed at my grandparents' house for two days every two to three weeks. I'm guessing that they each abused me approximately twice when I was there, whenever they found the opportunity. The maths is shocking, and I check and recheck my calculator. Three years, seventeen visits per year, two incidents per visit and two perpetrators – this adds up to 204 instances of abuse. As I make the calculations, my hands shake and my heart fills with empathy for little Martina. Placing my hand on my chest, I tell her she is safe now.

Later, I put fresh sheets and the summer doona on the bed to banish my nightmares. I sprinkle lavender oil onto the pillows. The scent hits my nostrils and reminds me that I've repeatedly rescued myself from the perpetrators, with patience, tenderness and self-compassion.

I hold anger in one hand and hope in the other. This is how I heal, one memory and flashback at a time, challenging two common and opposing societal expectations. The first is that victims of sexual violence will be forever damaged, and the second is that they can be completely healed, especially if they forgive their perpetrators. The truth lies somewhere in the middle. Holding anger in one hand and hope in the other allows me to care for my wounds tenderly, as a practical path towards healing. Yet healing is never perfect, nor is it achieved once and for all. And no, I have not forgiven the perpetrators who harmed me.

CHAPTER EIGHT

January 2015

We are still asleep when the phone rings.

'Hello, Martina. Your mother died an hour ago; her heart stopped,' my father tells me.

I gasp. I only talked with her yesterday before her back surgery. My mind whirls and I immediately think about having a drink. There's no alcohol in the house because I've been alcohol free for eight years, and Michael hasn't had a drink for twenty years.

'I thought her surgery went well?' I ask.

'I visited her yesterday afternoon and she seemed okay. Then her heart stopped in the night,' he replies.

'This is such a shock. Are you okay? Do you have someone there with you?' My blood is thumping loudly inside my ears.

'Yes, I'm okay. I'll let you know about the funeral. I have more calls to make now,' he says and hangs up.

I wake Michael and cry into his neck. He smells safe and familiar; his body is warm from sleep.

'My mum is dead,' I repeat over and over.

Michael holds me and rubs my back in circles while my cries become sobs. Now I'll never have a mum who hugs me tenderly.

'Let's book our flights.' Michael fetches his laptop while I blow my nose and think about who will be at the funeral, and that we'll have to pack our winter clothes since it's January and snowing in

Switzerland. I have a sneaky thought about the twenty-seven-hour flight where we'll be served free alcohol.

Just before eight in the morning, I park the car outside the grocery shop that also sells alcohol, wearing a singlet and track pants. My crying has subsided because I'm now single-minded about buying a bottle of vodka and getting a drink inside me. My craving is an arrow, and alcohol is the bullseye.

I check my face in the rearview mirror. My eyes are puffy from crying and my hair sticks up in several directions. I realise I forgot to put on a bra. It's going to be a hot January day. Intense heat already burns through the car windows and I try to fix my hair. The ABC news plays on the radio. There are bushfires in South Australia, and eight siblings, four girls and four boys, were found dead in a home in Cairns some weeks ago. Their mother stabbed them and is being held in a mental health facility in Brisbane.

I get out of the car, go into the shop and do a quick scan of the shelves. My hands shake with equal parts guilt and excitement. Today is the day I will cave and give myself permission to relapse.

'You only lose your mum once. You deserve a drink; it'll help soothe the pain,' the alcohol whispers in my ears.

I chit chat with Bruce the owner and pay with my debit card. He is a friendly local with a pockmarked face. He looks like he's just got out of bed too. I wonder whether he's judging me. He hasn't seen me buy alcohol for eight years. Back in the car, I unscrew the bottle top and take a couple of swigs of Vodka. A soothing warmth spreads through my chest and stomach. I call my brother Adrian.

'Hey, bro. Can you believe it? Mum's dead. Are you okay?' My voice is thick with unshed tears.

'I'm kind of numb.' Adrian's voice sounds far away.

I take another sip of vodka, hoping Adrian can't tell I'm drinking at eight in the morning.

'It's surreal, isn't it? If we do a eulogy, we'll have to try and come up with some positives about Mum,' I giggle, cheered by the alcohol as I swallow another mouthful.

'Yeah, I'd like to do a eulogy, but she was a hard woman.' Adrian laughs, but his voice is sad.

'I was talking to Mum yesterday before her surgery. She was so excited. She told me she was going to lose all the weight she'd put on and start exercising again,' I say, taking another sip of vodka.

'She was always on a diet, wasn't she?' Adrian chuckles.

§

Three days later, Lucie, Michael and I are standing around a small bar table in a private room of a fancy old castle on the outskirts of Basel. The walls are clad in expensive walnut, displaying oil paintings of old white men and snow-covered mountains. Michael and Lucie are drinking lemon, lime and bitters and I'm having a red wine. I watch as people move around the room at Mum's wake, taking polite sips of their wine. My head spins and I feel as if I'm split in two. Two selves collide in an astounding way: my childhood self, the one I don't want to think about, and my adult self, the one I somehow can't connect with.

I started drinking at ten this morning, with a couple of sips of brandy just before I stepped into the church for the funeral. I'd poured the brandy into an empty apple juice bottle and kept it in my handbag, taking small sips at regular intervals throughout the long, sad morning. While I don't want to be drunk, I want my pain to be numbed to just the right level. I try to remember the funeral, who spoke and what was said, but I've already forgotten. I look at the copy of my eulogy, but have no recollection now of what I said. I do remember there was music by Bach – a trio playing viola, cello and violin. Mum would have loved that.

'I'll stop drinking when we get back to Australia, I promise,' I tell Michael and Lucie, my face hot with shame. 'I know I've let you down.' I take their hands in mine for a few moments and make myself look into their eyes.

'It's okay. I know you'll stop, darling,' Michael says. He looks handsome in his dark suit and sky-blue shirt.

Lucie squeezes my hand. At fifteen, she is the youngest person here and she doesn't understand German. She busies herself texting her boyfriend back in Australia and I'm happy she's in love. Her eyes are wider than usual and she looks overwhelmed. I blame myself and my drinking. I gently kiss Lucie's forehead, holding my breath so she doesn't smell the alcohol. I say a silent prayer. *May I always strive to be a good-enough mother.*

As I stand holding onto the bar table, I take another sip of wine and watch the kaleidoscope of familiar faces. Distant relatives shake my hand and tell me they are sorry for my loss, that my eulogy was moving. I wrap Angelika, my childhood nanny, in a long embrace, then kiss her rosy cheeks three times, the Swiss way. How I love her. Everyone looks thirty years older, but still recognisable.

My childhood friend Lucie hugs Michael, Lucie and me. Her heart-shaped face and light blue eyes are so familiar, and I'm overwhelmed with gratefulness for all we've shared. She and her mother provided a safe haven for me, away from my unhappy family, when we were children. She holds me in her arms for a long time, her now middle-aged body soft and comforting.

'Your mum always frightened me. Even on the rare occasions we played at your house, her anger was like a storm waiting to break,' Lucie tells me. We stand with our arms wrapped around each other.

'Yeah, that's why we always played at your house. I'm so thankful for your friendship. You and your mum provided a sanctuary.' I hug

Lucie once more and feel her warmth and softness, so reminiscent of her mother.

I take a sip of wine and decide to check on my father, who's standing with his brother at a bar table across the room. He looks shorter, and when I hug him, his back and shoulders are stiff.

'Are you okay, Dad? The funeral was beautiful, wasn't it?' I fawn.

'It was a wonderful service, Martina. It is good to see so many people here who loved Susanne,' he says proudly.

As I stand next to him, I reflect that only a few days ago I was a sober woman, committed to handling my emotions like an adult. How quickly alcohol has hijacked my brain. I'm dismayed that this overwhelming craving has returned after all this time; I'd been convinced I would never want to drink again. As I stand next to my father, alcohol, the trickster, sits on my shoulder and whispers to me, 'Go on, drink as much as you want, Martina. You deserve it. After all, your mum just died.'

We're a mere few kilometres away from the house where I was abused as a small child. I have another mouthful of wine, push away my memories and decide to think instead about how blessed I am by our family of three – Michael, Lucie and me. I can't wait to get on the plane to return to our real lives in Australia – to reclaim my sobriety and the life I've painstakingly built so far away from my Swiss childhood.

Later, Adrian and I quietly share memories of Mum.

'I always worried she'd kill herself,' Adrian says sadly.

'Me too. I wonder why we never talked about this when we were kids.' I pick at my nails.

'Yes, we each suffered alone.' Adrian gazes into the distance.

I reflect that my brothers and I had to carry our emotional burdens alone, like heavy backpacks filled with rocks. Together, Adrian and I gaze out the window at the winter landscape and the steely grey sky. Although we've survived our childhood, we continue to be affected by our early wounding. And yet, how healing it is to sit and talk together like this, after five decades of silence.

CHAPTER NINE

2019

On a winter's day, I drink my morning coffee and gaze at the teeming rain outside the sliding doors. The heater ticks and I think about Mum, who's been gone for four years now. I remember the day I viewed her body in the cold morgue. She was lying in an open coffin and dressed from head to toe in beige; even her soft leather slip-on shoes were beige. I wonder who chose her outfit. It wasn't her best colour, especially with the pallor of death. I leaned forward and kissed her forehead, which was as cold and hard as cement. I gave a small scream with the shock of how dead she was. Her beautiful hands were still elegant as I stroked their tapestry of blue veins. She looked just like Mum, but death had already carried her to that other place, not reachable by the living.

I hope she's at peace, reunited and laughing with her cousins and girlfriends. Most of all, I hope she hasn't run into her father or brother, the paedophiles from her childhood. But I'm certain they are in the hell realm, while she's in a merry heaven of good food and laughter, together with her friends who loved her deeply.

I wish I could let her know that I relapsed with alcohol when she died because I was stricken by a profound and unexpected grief, realising I'd never have a mother who told me she loved me, hugged me tenderly, or told me she was proud of me.

She was a terrible mother but I love her, nonetheless. I no longer carry the pain of being unmothered because I learned to mother myself as an adult by attending therapy and having my own child whom I adore and parent with gentleness and respect.

Regaining my sobriety after returning to Australia is one of the greatest blessings I've received. Grateful for this second, hard-won sobriety, I'm proud that at least I didn't relapse with pills when Mum died. Pills were a much harder habit to kick. I'd been Mum's secret apprentice in self-medicating and learned by watching her soothe her pain with the various boxes and bottles of tablets from the red medicine cabinet above the toilet. I started stealing her pills when I was twelve. Like her, I swallowed pills to soothe the curse of being an unloved and abused child.

I wonder whether Mum ever tried to give up using pills. I wish we could have talked together about our reliance on the magical yellow, white and pink tablets. Perhaps we could have even helped each other to break free of them. When I finally had the courage to give them up in my thirties, I walked the floors of the house for four sleepless nights, my restless legs unbearable. My legs jerked and quivered, cramped and flailed – a typical sign of opioid withdrawal. The only thing to do was to keep walking, so I paced all night. As I walked through the house, I cried quietly, not wanting to wake Michael and too ashamed to tell him how much Mersyndol and Valium I'd been taking. Like Mum, I used to pop three Valium in one go and welcomed the blessed arrival of soft fuzziness within half an hour. Pills made me feel safe, unharmed by people and events, unafraid of making mistakes or being rejected. Pills protected my heart from hurt, or so I believed. I know they similarly helped Mum when she couldn't help herself another way.

There is a remaining sense of sadness that Mum never got to study medicine or work outside the home after she married. She was depressed and unfulfilled as a housewife, while I had the opportunity to study in my late twenties and earn three degrees. Going to university changed my life's trajectory, guiding me toward purpose and deeply fulfilling work. What a long way I've come since being a sex worker who was dependent on a guru. Finally, I believe in my own worth. I wish Mum could have had the opportunity to study and work as a doctor outside the home. I'm certain she would have been happier if she could have used her fierce intelligence to help others.

I also reflect on the hatred Mum and I shared for our unruly female bodies. Mum was dieting well into her late eighties.

'Dieting is the most potent political sedative in women's history. A quietly mad population is a tractable one,' Naomi Wolfe wrote in the 1990s.

I wish I could have talked to Mum about her mistrust of her body. The diet industry is worth seventy billion dollars each year. While Mum and I stepped on scales and thought about the calories we consumed, we didn't have to weep over the terrible betrayal of being abused by our male relatives. Pulling an old photo album from the bookshelf, I look at pictures of myself in adolescence and observe a beautiful young woman with a natural, sweet and curvy body. While Mum and I were busy hating our bodies, we remained straightjacketed in female obedience. Dad and the boys never had to think about their weight. In our family, dieting and body shame were reserved exclusively for Mum and me, because we were born female.

If Mum was still alive, I would take her out to an Italian restaurant, where we would order triple-cheese pizza, gorgonzola gnocchi, garlic bread infused with the finest olive oil and several calorie-rich desserts including tiramisu, zabaglione and cannoli.

Wherever Mum is now, I know she no longer needs pills or diets to soothe her aching heart. Her spirit is whole and healed. A feeling of forgiveness towards Mum suffuses my body. I love to think she is finally at peace. In my mind, I reach out and hold her beautiful hands and stroke them gently. I kiss her cheeks three times, the Swiss way, but with warmth.

CHAPTER TEN

2022

My father is a tiny ninety-six-year-old man pulling a small brown suitcase, a grey rucksack on his back. I watch him as he nimbly rushes towards us at our arranged meeting spot at the Zurich train station.

'Hi, Dad, how are you?' I hug him.

His back is stiff with arthritis, and I take in his musty old man smell. The left lapel and pant leg of his blue corduroy suit are covered with food stains.

'Hallo, Martina. Hallo, Michael.' He shakes Michael's hand. 'We must rush to platform twelve to catch the train,' he declares in his brisk German accent.

My heart hammers inside my chest and I wish I were no longer vulnerable to this remote man of my childhood. Michael and I have travelled to Switzerland to spend time with him. Trains arrive and leave, and the departure of our train to the mountains is announced over the loudspeaker in three languages, German, French and Italian.

Michael and I hurry behind my dad, barely able to keep up with this spry, elderly man. As we run behind him, Michael nudges me and winks, encouraging me to see the humour in my dad's brisk interaction with us, even though we haven't seen him for several years. We are going to be spending three days together walking in the mountains. When we locate platform twelve and enter the train, we find three seats in the already crowded carriage. A young man sits across from me, while Dad faces Michael who is sitting next to me.

As soon as we've taken our seats, my father speaks loudly.

'I have achieved so much in my fortunate life. I want to give back to Switzerland, my motherland. I owe her a great debt.' His voice booms, and I'm worried that everyone in the crowded carriage can hear every word.

'I'm glad to hear that.' I tap my right foot with irritation.

'I have made so much money and have had such success that I will donate a large sum to the university for research. I built my wealth from nothing, from sheer determination and hard work. Now it is time to give back,' he continues, clearly proud of himself.

I wonder about his three children and three grandchildren and what we mean to him. He still hasn't asked about us. Inwardly rolling my eyes, my right leg is now pumping up and down rapidly. I make eye contact with the young man sitting across from me and mouth a 'sorry' that he must listen to my father's bragging. His sense of pride and his craving for admiration are embarrassing. While not malevolent, he carries an irritating air of self-importance.

'I had such a wonderful job at the Swiss pharmaceutical company where I worked my whole life. Now I will put my money back into important research,' he continues loudly, as if he wants the whole carriage to hear.

Through the train window, the city of Zurich recedes, soon replaced by green meadows where cows graze, large brass bells hanging around their necks. Wooden farmhouses, hundreds of years old, fly past.

§

The following day, we hike in the mountains near the village of Chandolin, where we once spent childhood holidays, two thousand metres above sea level. The air is crisp, and the mountains surround us like steady friends. In childhood, they were snow-capped all year round, but now they are green; the snow has melted due to global warming.

As we walk together, I think about the three men who each crushed me in their own way when I was a child. My grandfather and uncle physically crushed me, while my father crushed my spirit with his indifference. When he found out about my sexual abuse when I was in my late twenties, his silence was deeply hurtful. I went to the letterbox every day and waited two long months to hear from him. When he finally wrote, he suggested he could pay for my therapy, which was not what I wanted from him.

Instead, I needed him to show empathy for the harm that had been done to me. I was the forgotten child, taken to my grand-parents' home on weekends, while my parents and brothers went on European holidays without me. Despite obvious signs, Mum and Dad didn't care to notice that I was being sexually abused by my uncle and grandfather. Instead, they chose to look the other way. As a small child, I lived in constant fear of men.

Dad hated Mum's father and brother. As we walk in the mountains, I wonder why he thought it was okay for me to be regularly left with them without protection. Dad and Mum were culpable by omission, neglecting to shield me from harm. I never felt loved by Dad, never felt he was interested in me. To safeguard my emotional wellbeing, I learned to withdraw from my family.

§

Later, while walking along a meandering creek, I decide to focus on self-care, taking my negative focus off my father, whom I cannot change. No longer willing to give my power to him, I decide to soothe my anger and hurt through the deliberate practice of self-compassion.

'May I be peaceful, may I be patient, may I be grateful, may I be healed,' I whisper silently.

I focus on a self-soothing exercise I learned in therapy: five things I am grateful for, four things I see, three things I hear, two things I feel touching my skin and one thing I like about myself.

I'm grateful for Michael's steadfast presence, for having an authentic and loving bond with Lucie, for nourishing friendships, for my good health and for the natural beauty all around me.

I gaze at the small pink mountain flowers, the little creek we traverse, the majestic mountains and the fragrant pine trees.

I hear my father drone on but quickly dismiss this. Instead, I focus on the gurgling sound of the creek, the buzzing of bees and the gentle thud of our footsteps.

I sense the softness of my woollen jumper against my neck and wrists and the grass, gravel and rock beneath my feet.

Proud of my ability to recover from the past, I give thanks for this opportunity to heal. I repeat the mindfulness exercise many times, while Dad continues his monologue.

I also breathe in to the count of four and out to the count of six. These are the tools I learned from Robbie to help regulate my emotions, tools that have become my abiding, reliable friends.

'I'm a wealthy man and have achieved so much more than I ever hoped,' Dad intrudes.

Michael and I need not reply. When we sit down to rest on a log, I create a small work of ephemeral art out of pine needles and cones, small sticks and leaves. It becomes a friendly mountain creature, and as I build it, I experience a delicious inner peace. My stomach and neck relax, and we share a block of hazelnut chocolate, savouring its sweet crunchiness. We walk on while I feel strangely calm, knowing I can't change my father.

That night, as we eat dinner at a restaurant, Dad continues his stream of consciousness. My throat is tight as I decide to speak the truth.

'Dad, I need to tell you how I feel. I want you to listen and not interrupt me, please. In childhood, adulthood and even now during our time together, I've felt unheard and unseen by you. This really hurts my heart. I feel very sad that we have no real connection.'

Once I start talking, my voice gains strength.

'I do listen to you,' he says dismissively. His gaze shifts around the restaurant, scanning the people at the other tables.

'No, you don't. Every time I speak, you interrupt and continue with your stories of success. It brings back the painful reminder that you weren't there for my brothers and me in childhood. You chose to ignore the sexual abuse I endured. While you weren't the perpetrator, I do hold you and Mum culpable by omission.' My voice has become plaintive.

'That is very unfortunate,' Dad says drily. 'Let's order dessert now.' He waves his right hand to summon the waiter.

'Dad, you've just done it again. You've not listened to me. As your daughter, I'm just so sad.' I cross my arms in irritation.

Dad nods, non-committal.

We order dessert and I devour it rapidly, squashing my pain. Michael puts his hand on my thigh to show his support as my right leg pumps up and down beneath the table. What a comfort he is. *How have I managed to choose such a good man*, I wonder gratefully.

An unintended benefit of spending time with my father is that I'm able to gain greater compassion for my mother. It must have been heartbreaking for her to feel unloved by a husband who didn't have room for anyone but himself. His focus was always on becoming wealthier and more successful, yet he never gave her enough money to buy groceries and other necessities. He showed her no affection and always chose work over his wife and children. I understand now why Mum cried so often about her loveless marriage.

Deeply grateful that Michael and I have built a stable and love-filled marriage, I embrace this hard-won equilibrium. Michael's calming presence grounds and soothes me. That night, we lie in bed in our hotel room, and I'm astonished by all the sorrows that have passed and the countless precious gifts that have come to me. We giggle together about the mad comedy of our day with my father, who will never change.

CHAPTER ELEVEN

2022

I make up Lucie's bed, put fresh flowers on her bedside table and place a rolled towel at the foot of her bed. I've been in a state of excitement all day because Lucie's coming from Sydney to stay for the weekend.

She walks through the front door in the early evening, and we both scream with joy.

'Mama!' she yells.

'Noonie!' I shout.

'I've missed you so much,' I say as we hug, and I breathe in her familiar smell.

'Mum, look at my hair! I paid a hundred and fifty dollars to go blonde, and now it's purple. I hate it.' She plonks herself down on the sofa.

'It looks really cool,' I say, as I stroke her hair.

We sit on the sofa, drinking tea. We touch forefinger to forefinger, very delicately, barely moving. What a sacred moment. Then, a little later, we touch palms, once again very lightly. I no longer have permission to smoosh her face between my hands or to give her loud kisses, which she readily consented to as a four-year-old. No more raspberry kisses on her chubby baby stomach.

She's an independent twenty-three-year-old, separate from me, and I truly respect that. She works as a social worker in a women's refuge and has been passionate about feminism and social justice for over a decade. Lucie is no longer like a puppy who loves my abundant demonstrations of affection. Now I treat her a little like a deer – one that I must approach tentatively, gently, always respecting her boundaries, allowing her to lead the mother-daughter dance, and letting her come to me. I'm grateful I'm not like my mother, who would criticise me the moment I walked through the door, even after a year's absence.

'Your hair looks cheap and brassy. You're fat. You stink of cigarettes. You'll die an early death from lung cancer.' This is what she used to say to me in her harshest German.

This is why I know I must practise restraint in the way I speak to Lucie. By doing so, I show respect for her autonomy.

§

Later that night, dressed in our pyjamas, we lie on Lucie's bed. Reggie is stretched out on his back between us, his legs up in the air. He trusts us, and we talk to him in baby talk, rubbing his stomach and gently scratching him behind his ears.

'Mum, I've started to hate men. Not Dad or Gabe, but all the men who inflict a thousand harms against women.' Lucie sounds sad.

I nod and lightly stroke her hair. I feel guilty that I've probably taught her to hate men.

'You don't really like men either, do you, Mum?' Lucie asks me.

'I do like Dad, Bill your godfather, your boyfriend Gabe and your uncle Adrian. That's four men,' I laugh.

Lucie tells me about her work at the women's refuge, where she constantly witnesses women and children who've been harmed by men in the most horrific and degrading ways.

'I feel disgusted by men,' Lucie sighs and pats Reggie's stomach while he groans contentedly.

'I understand, darling. In my work over the past thirty years,

215

I've seen countless women suffer at the hands of men.' I stroke her forehead and push her hair off her face.

'How do you deal with it, Mum? It's so hard.' Lucie looks exhausted already, at such a young age.

'We're lucky to have amazing jobs where we can make a difference in women and children's lives,' I tell her.

We discuss the one hundred women who lost their lives to their male partners and ex-partners this year, the fact that one in four women and children experience domestic violence, and the frustrating reality that these statistics are largely ignored.

'We have to take very good care of ourselves so that we can continue to do our work,' I say, smelling Reggie's fur and kissing the soft blond curls on the top of his head.

I continue to lightly stroke Lucie's hair, which is indeed purple.

'Lucie, I'm so proud of you,' I tell her. 'Do you think your job is too overwhelming for someone so young?'

'No, I love it, Mum. I'm so glad I can make a difference.' She rubs her tired eyes.

Being Lucie's mum has been an immense gift. When I think about how I followed the guru's instructions by having myself sterilised at twenty-five, I feel so fortunate that I was able to have the sterilisation reversed. The moment she was born, I knew I'd never intentionally harm her, and it appears I've been a trustworthy, though not faultless, mum.

As we lie together on her bed, I say a silent prayer of gratitude for Lucie. Her name means 'bearer of light'. How much light she brings to her friends, family, Michael and me. As an adult, she brings this same warm beam to the women and children she helps in her work.

Lucie's eyes are closed, and she's fallen asleep. I watch her face and marvel at the two precious dimples on her left cheek. As I listen to her even breaths, I am filled with gladness that my daughter still wants to come home. I kiss her forehead, turn off the bedside light and leave her bedroom door ajar, just as I did when she was a little girl. Reggie remains stretched out on his back beside her and takes a long, contented sigh.

EPILOGUE

2025

Today I reflect on everything I learned since leaving the guru thirty-five years ago. Attending therapy in my late twenties helped me understand that no one would come and save me. I'm the one who must rescue myself, by doing the slow, painstaking work of admitting the truth about my past. To heal, I had to find the courage and patience to listen to my inner child's sorrow and care for her wounds tenderly and consistently.

I've had to accept that there are no shortcuts and that healing is much messier and slower than I could ever have imagined. I've journeyed like a turtle on the path of recovery. This sacred inner work has entailed many setbacks that required grit and perseverance. I've stumbled and fallen, again and again. However, each time I fall, I stand back up, like a toddler learning to walk. Sometimes I stay down for hours, or even a couple of days, before I find the will to rise again. It has taken guts to grieve my story of violence at the hands of those who should have protected me, while the rest of my family looked the other way. I've had to face the full impact of what my perpetrators did to me. They nearly ruined me. Yet I have survived.

An important truth I learned along the way is that we can't heal in isolation. Recovery requires us to share our stories of shame and brokenness. I've been fortunate to find a partner and safe friends who have consistently supported me on my journey of falling apart and mending. They tell me, 'I believe you.' They ask me, 'How can

I support you?' When I talk to Michael about my childhood, he hugs me gently and validates my sorrow. 'I'm so sorry you weren't loved the way you deserved,' he tells me.

These words of care have gradually transformed my suffering into a kind of 'radical acceptance', meaning accepting the unacceptable, a term coined by the psychiatrist Marsha Linehan. I've come to accept that I'll never be able to go back in time and have a happy childhood. Instead, I acknowledge that I grew up in a dysfunctional family system from which I must rescue myself daily.

Aged sixty, I know I must show up and care for myself by tending to my wounds. I build a routine of walks with my dog, being in nature, going to the gym, having afternoon naps, reading voraciously, laughing with my women friends and, of course, spending time with my family.

'I'll do whatever it takes to heal,' I whisper when I wake from a nightmare about the past. Sometimes I still try to lock my painful memories inside a box and throw away the key, but I accept that's not how it works. I must be courageous and look every instance of harm in the face. Lovingly, I take my memories out of their box and hold them gently and with reverence, like tiny baby birds. Softly, I stroke them. I no longer expect a guru to save me from myself. While I accept responsibility for my life, I also know the sexual abuse and other harms I suffered were not my fault.

When I was a child, I loved the adults who abused me, which in turn caused me to love the guru who used his devotees for his own gains. I only saw this truth in my late twenties, when my prefrontal cortex had fully developed and I was finally strong enough to break free from the guru. At long last, I learned to stand on my own two feet.

I recently read a book by Steve Taylor, *The Leap*. He argues that the psychological neediness of the devotee is the key to understanding her dependence on a guru. We may turn to spiritual teachers with a genuine desire for growth, but this longing becomes entangled with a deeper, more troubling urge – the desire to return to a childlike state of surrender and dependency.

According to Taylor, instead of guiding followers toward true awakening, the guru becomes the centre of a dynamic that hinders growth and encourages emotional regression. The feeling of bliss or unity that a devotee experiences is akin to the early bond between an infant and its mother. The guru, cast as a flawless being, is placed beyond reproach. No matter how lavish his lifestyle – millions of dollars, fleets of luxury cars, armed guards – or how demeaning his treatment of followers, his actions are excused, just as a child might defend an abusive parent.

As I reflect on this, with the benefit of maturity and critical thinking, I'm stunned by the blind devotion I once offered the guru who exploited his followers for sex, power and wealth. At the same time, I hold compassion for the young woman I was back then – a nineteen-year-old survivor of trauma, shaped by childhood abuse, my wounds deepened by the sex work that echoed my early experiences.

I didn't yet understand that my worth extended far beyond my body. And though I was foolish, I admire young Martina's determination to seek healing, even if the path I chose was painfully flawed. Grateful to be free of my former dependence on the guru, I stand firmly on my own two feet – an adult able to think critically and care for myself.

§

When I got into the University of Sydney in my late twenties, I sat in lecture theatres and suffered panic attacks. Everyone was intelligent, while I was too stupid to succeed at tertiary education. Over time though, being a university student empowered me to think deeply, allowing me to work in a field that has continued to be profoundly meaningful for thirty years. Attending university opened many doors that were previously closed to me. Above all, tertiary education empowered me to be of service to others. I developed self-confidence and earned three degrees. For the first time in my life, I genuinely believed in my own intelligence and worth.

In 2014, I completed a PhD titled 'Women of Courage' on the topic of sexual assault and the legal system. I chose this subject matter because in my work I've witnessed on countless occasions how the legal system betrays women and children who've suffered sexual violence. As a therapist working in government sexual assault services, and later in private practice as a contractor for the Attorney-General's Department, I've had the honour of accompanying countless survivors of sexual assault and domestic violence on their sacred journeys of recovery. This has been my passion for three decades. I've also lectured on this and other topics at the University of Newcastle for the past twelve years.

The healing I've received enables me to offer hope to my clients who feel broken, just as I did thirty-five years ago when I first started attending therapy. I tell my clients it won't always feel this painful, that there is hope even in the darkest of times. By being believed and supported, and by learning skills that empower and heal, they slowly, sometimes imperceptibly, recover.

Every time I consider the statistics on sexual violence in Australia, my blood thumps loudly inside my ears. One in four girls and women, and one in seven boys and men, experience sexual violence. When I teach in a lecture theatre, about one hundred students usually attend. This means that twenty-five women and fourteen men attending the lecture have suffered sexual assault. I look out at my students from the lectern and want to weep. How brave they are!

Research has found that less than thirteen per cent of victims report to police, and only 1.4 per cent of offenders are convicted in court. In a recent study by the University of New South Wales, one in six men admit to being sexually attracted to children under the age of fourteen, and one in ten admit to having sexually abused a child. I hope these statistics make you, my dear readers, angry.

§

One of my heroines and a pioneer in the field of interpersonal violence is the psychiatrist, Judith Herman, whom Robbie introduced me to. She has helped me in my recovery more than any other expert and writer. Her book *Trauma and Recovery* has remained my favourite text throughout my career. Here is one of the most important truths that Judith Herman wrote in 1992:

> His most consistent feature is his apparent normality. How much more comforting it would be if the perpetrator were easily recognisable, obviously deviant and disturbed. His demeanor provides an excellent camouflage, for few people believe that extraordinary crimes can be committed by men of such conventional appearance.

Indeed, my two perpetrators appeared to be normal men. They were highly regarded by society, a judge and a politician. But behind closed doors, when no one was watching, they turned into dangerous, greedy monsters.

Herman has been a guiding light on my path of healing. She states that recovery must always be based on the empowerment of the survivor, which can occur only in the context of safe relationships. Robbie helped me discover my power, reduce isolation, diminish the helplessness I experienced and increase my range of choices. She deliberately and consistently countered the dynamics of dominance in the therapeutic relationship. She bore witness to the crimes that had been committed against me and always affirmed a position of solidarity with me.

Herman's three stages of healing allowed me to build a life of purpose and compassion. The first stage is to create safety. This included restoring control, self-care, establishing a safe environment, addressing eating and sleeping, and reducing hyperarousal and other symptoms of trauma. It took me several years to establish safety and self-care when I first started my work with Robbie. This meant learning to feed myself three meals a day, like a good mother would, instead of allowing myself only one measly evening meal. It meant stopping smoking my much-loved Alpine cigarettes and giving up pills and alcohol to numb my pain. This took time and entailed several relapses and setbacks.

The second stage involved remembrance and mourning. Herman describes that during this stage, the survivor tells her story, leading to grief and eventual integration. Sharing my story required immense courage, and I often feared that Robbie wouldn't believe me. Given how horrific my experiences were, and that the topic of sexual abuse wasn't yet openly discussed in the 1980s, I worried she might think I was lying. Instead, Robbie always offered a steady, compassionate presence in the face of my suffering.

In the third stage, I learned to reconnect with everyday life. This entailed finding the courage to walk away from the guru and my cult family, and step into the world of ordinary life. Having come to terms with the trauma of the past, I faced the task of creating a better future and gradually built a life filled with connection and meaning. I was fortunate to find a partner, safe friends and several family members who have supported me consistently and lovingly.

The progression through Herman's three stages is arduous. Not everyone reaches the goal of recovery. Many are tragically lost along the way to addiction, mental illness, self-harm and suicide.

§

Questions remain. For example, can we ever come to terms with the countless crimes committed against women and children? More importantly, how can we put an end to domestic and sexual violence? Violence prevention must always be our most urgent task. The government continues to underfund and largely ignore the urgent crisis of homicide and violence against women and children.

Frequently enraged when I sit with vulnerable clients, I'm grateful for my rage. I consider it my superpower. It allows me to cope with the countless women and children who have sat and wept on the couch in my counselling room. If I had a bucket to catch all the tears my clients have shed over thirty years, it would be overflowing, the tears covering the office floor. My tears mingle with those of my clients' and our grief-soaked tissues would fill a large green wheelie bin. My own experience of childhood trauma fuels my passion to help others. My anger gives me the energy and commitment required to help those who have suffered interpersonal harm. Holding anger in one hand and hope in the other, these two powerful emotions steer me each day, both in my work and in my personal life.

ACKNOWLEDGEMENTS

There are countless people I'm deeply grateful for, starting with the women from childhood who provided succour and kindness. My primary school teacher Fraulein Beckmann, my nanny Angelika Herzog, my dearest friend Lucie and her mum Frau Heidi Koechlin, my godmother Christine Gross-Gerwig and most of all, my dear aunt Vera Zuercher-Gerwig, who has unconditionally supported me and who was the first to say she believed me when I disclosed the sexual abuse.

My deepest gratitude to Robbie Corbett, the steadfast guide who walked alongside me, taught me to care for myself with tenderness and always believed in me, even when I didn't.

Big thanks to my brother Adrian Zangger and his wife Paula Zangger, whose kindness and unwavering care mean the world to me. Adrian, we grew up together in that frightening and joyless home and we experienced many of the same sorrows. May we continue to heal.

I'm grateful for the generous readers of my early, messy drafts, including Lisa Frazer, Cath Napier, Maya Drew, Sharon Unie, Marika Polemis and Tori Montague.

I give special thanks to my sister refugees from the cult of Rajneesh: Jo-anne McGowan, Patricia Austin, Anne Reessing and Elizabeth Gunn. We made it out of there!

With extra big gratitude to my writing mentor, Chloe Higgins, who helped me lay down the weight of academia and step into the wild beauty of creative writing. You urged me to dive deep, to write with rawness and courage.

Heartfelt thanks to my publisher Jane Curry of Ventura Press, for believing in both me and this story from the beginning. Thank you to my editors Kate Cuthbert and Amanda Hemmings, whose steady insight and assured guidance shaped this book into something far stronger.

My profoundest thanks go to my husband Michael Page and our daughter Lucie Zangger-Page. Your warmth, humour and loving kindness have brought a stability and joy I could never have dreamt of. I'm a much better person with you in my life. Thank you for your patience, especially when I was cranky, preoccupied, menopausal and lost in the world of writing this story.

REFERENCES

Hall, E., *Made of Rivers*, Self-published, 2023

Herman, J. L., *Trauma and Recovery: The aftermath of violence – from domestic abuse to political terror*, Basic Books, 1992

Holloway, A., *The Bipolar Bear Family: When a Parent Has Bipolar Disorder*, Author House, 2006

McKay, M., Rogers, P. D., & McKay, J., *When Anger Hurts Your Relationship: 10 simple solutions for couples who fight*. New Harbinger Publications, 1999

Osho, *My Way: The way of the white clouds*, Rajneesh Foundation, 1978

Osho, *The Book of Secrets: 112 meditations to discover the mystery within*, St. Martin's Griffin, 1974

Osho, *Commune: A hope for humanity*, Rebel Publishing House, 1987

Osho, *The Dhammapada: The way of the Buddha*, (Vol. 3), Rajneesh Foundation, 1979

Osho, *The Book of Understanding: Creating your own path to freedom*, Harmony Books, 2006

Osho, *Creativity: Unleashing the forces within*, St. Martin's Griffin, 2001

Osho, *Love, Freedom, Aloneness: The koan of relationships*, St. Martin's Griffin, 2002

Osho, *The Book of Women: Why has woman been so repressed?*, Rebel Publishing House, 1999

Taylor, S., *The Leap: The psychology of spiritual awakening*, Hay House, UK, 2017

Wolfe N., *The Beauty Myth: How images of beauty are used against women*, William Morrow and Company, 1991

www.ingramcontent.com/pod-product-compliance
Lightning Source LLC
Chambersburg PA
CBHW021800190326
41518CB00007B/378